Menstrual Cramps
Self Help Book

Dr. Susan Lark's

Menstrual Cramps
Self Help Book

Susan Lark, M.D.

*Effective solutions for pain and discomfort
due to menstrual cramps and PMS*

CELESTIALARTS
Berkeley, California

Katherine —
I hope this
helps in some
way —
Love you —
mom

To my wonderful husband Jim and
my darling daughter Rebecca.
To the health and well-being of all women.

NOTE: The information in this book is meant to complement the advice and guidance of your physician, not replace it. It is very important that women with menstrual cramps have this problem evaluated by a physician. If you are under the care of a physician, you should discuss any major changes in your regimen with him or her. Because this is a book and not a medical consultation, keep in mind that the information presented here may not apply in your particular case. Whenever a question arises, discuss it with your physician.

CELESTIAL ARTS
P.O. Box 7123, Berkeley, CA 94707

Cover design by Fifth Street Design
Text design and composition by Brad Greene
Photographs by Ronald May
Illustrations by Shelley Reeves Smith

Library of Congress Cataloging-in-Publication Data
Lark, Susan M., 1945-
    [Menstrual cramps self help book]
    Dr. Susan Lark's The menstrual cramps self help book : effective solutions
for pain and discomfort due to menstrual cramps and PMS / Susan Lark.
        p.   cm.
    Includes index.
    ISBN 0-89087-771-8
    1. Dysmenorrhea--Popular works.   I. Title.
RG181.L373 1995
618-1'72--dc20
                                                                95-14861
                                                                CIP

Contents

Introduction: A Self Help Approach to Menstrual Cramps   1

Part I: Identifying the Problem

Chapter 1   What Are Menstrual Cramps?   9

Part II: Evaluating Your Symptoms

Chapter 2   The Menstrual Cramps Workbook   21

Part III: Finding the Solution

Chapter 3   The Menstrual Cramps Self Help Program—
             Complete Treatment Chart   61

Chapter 4   Dietary Principles for Menstrual Cramps   63

Chapter 5   Menus, Meal Plans & Recipes   83

Chapter 6   Vitamins, Minerals & Herbs for
             Menstrual Cramps   107

Chapter 7   Stress Reduction for Menstrual Cramps   131

Chapter 8   Breathing Exercises for Menstrual Cramps   145

Chapter 9   Physical Exercise for Menstrual Cramps   153

Chapter 10   Yoga for Menstrual Cramps   169

Chapter 11   Acupressure for Menstrual Cramps   183

Chapter 12   Treating Menstrual Cramps with Drugs   199

Chapter 13   How to Put Your Program Together   205

Index   211

Introduction

A Self Help Approach to Menstrual Cramps

I have been a physician practicing women's health care and preventive medicine for almost two decades in the San Francisco area. I have worked with many thousands of women, combining the traditional medical diagnostic and therapeutic techniques with a strong emphasis on the important role that a healthy lifestyle plays in promoting wellness and preventing disease.

Helping so many women gain relief from their health-care problems has been a truly wonderful and satisfying experience. In my medical practice, I have always emphasized information and education on self-care along with any medical treatments given. I have always wanted my patients to be knowledgeable participants in their own health-care program. I have never failed to be impressed with how positively my patients have responded to this approach. My women patients have uniformly communicated to me that they have an intense desire for information on how to stay healthy and symptom-free. They also understand how important it is for them to take an active role in their own healing process. I personally encountered the need for information during my teenage years and throughout my twenties when I suffered from severe menstrual cramps and PMS. It was only after I started my own self-care program that I finally got permanent relief from these problems.

Learning to Cure My Own Menstrual Cramps

My own experience with menstrual cramps was a long and agonizing one. I began to have severe cramps as soon as I started to menstruate as a young teenager. I found very few treatment options available to me as a teen, except for aspirin, a hot water bottle, or simply going to bed and lying there for hours in pain, hoping the cramps would finally stop. Very little information was available on self-care treatments at that time, and I received absolutely no lifestyle information from my physician on the importance of nutrition and exercise in preventing cramps.

My cramps continued to be quite severe throughout college and medical school. As a doctor-in-training, I had access to the best medical care. I tried every medication possible that might help me—pain pills, muscle relaxants, and antispasmodics—but nothing really helped relieve my symptoms effectively, except on a very temporary basis. I also suffered from PMS during those years, so my menstrual cramps were preceded by days of anxiety, irritability, bloating, and food cravings. It is no wonder that I regarded menstruation with a feeling of apprehension. I still remember episodes of menstrual cramps severe enough to compel me to leave the hospital ward when I was a medical student. I would go to the medical students' on-call room and suffer through the agony of viselike cramps.

Luckily, during my internship year, my situation changed. I was doing my specialty training in obstetrics and gynecology and spent quite a bit of time reading the new medical research in this field. By chance, I spotted an article on the use of nutrition to treat breast cysts in an obstetrics and gynecology journal. I had never been exposed to the concept of nutrition as therapy before; in fact, it had never occurred to me that what I ate could affect my health status. I was intrigued by the article, which described the successful treatment of breast lumps with the use of vitamins. I began to spend time in the medical library looking for information on the treatment of menstrual disorders through nutrition.

During the next few years, I began to test a simple self-care program on myself. I made some dietary changes, cutting out sugar, fat, and caffeine, which had been the mainstay of my diet. As a busy medical student, I had depended on "fast foods" such as cola drinks, coffee, sweet rolls, and ham sandwiches to help me stay awake and provide a quick source of energy during busy late nights taking care of sick patients. I started to cut down on my junk-food intake, and I began to eat more whole grains, fresh vegetables, and fruits. I started myself on a vitamin and mineral program that I put together based on my study of the research in nutritional medicine.

I was amazed with the results. My symptoms, which had plagued me for years, began to diminish on a month-by-month basis. My quality of life improved as my symptoms receded in a dramatic way.

I began to exercise more regularly and started to learn about and practice stress management techniques. I felt better than I ever had in my life. After several years of self-care, my symptoms were entirely gone and have never come back.

For the past eighteen years my menstrual periods have been painless and symptom-free. I am now in my late forties and have had years of my periods coming and going without interfering with my life. In fact, they are so comfortable that I never know when they are going to start, except for the fact that I keep a menstrual calendar. I am planning to have an equally comfortable menopause when that phase of my life begins.

Learning to Help My Patients

I was my first successful menstrual-cramp-and-PMS patient. In the years since I put together my own treatment program, I have worked with many thousands of women patients who have benefited from a self-care approach. I have spent years researching the use of diet, nutrition, and many other lifestyle techniques that benefit health and help to prevent disease. I have learned specific acupressure points, yoga stretches, exercise routines, and many stress management techniques in order to offer my patients many different self-care options. My goal with patients has always been to give them the information, education, and resources to help them become healthier women and then maintain this state through healthy lifestyle practices. Researchers have made many advances in drug treatment. Today there are medications for menstrual cramps to which I never had access as a teenager. Many of these treat the symptoms of menstrual cramps very effectively. In my practice I use medications, too, for those women who need immediate symptomatic relief. My patients today do not have to wait years, as I did, to see their symptoms diminish. Most of them feel much better within one or two menstrual cycles.

How to Use This Book

There are many women in different parts of the United States whom I will obviously never see as patients in my medical practice. I feel strongly that any woman interested in self-care should have access to this information. So I wrote this book to share with women the self-care techniques that I have found to be most useful through many years of medical practice. All this self help information is now available in this book, and I hope you will find it as useful as my patients have.

I continue to practice these techniques, too. Preventive health care has had tremendous benefits for me; I am healthier and more productive now than I was ten years ago. I plan to feel better and to be even healthier ten years from now. I am continually expanding my own knowledge about self help and am constantly researching new health-care techniques for menstrual cramps and low back pain.

The menstrual cramp and low back pain self help program provides very important information for all women suffering from these problems. I have written the program so that each woman reading this book can select from a wide variety of self help treatment options that I have included. A treatment plan that utilizes only one method and purports to be the only treatment for menstrual cramps and low back pain will probably work for only a small percentage of women. In my own medical practice, I have found that results are much better if I completely individualize each patient's treatment program. By overlapping treatments from various disciplines, most women find combinations that work for them. You will be able to find a combination that works for you, too.

After seeing so many of my patients become healthier over time, I am a firm believer in the power of self-care. Changing lifestyle habits in a beneficial way gives the body a chance to heal itself. I don't believe that an unfavorable medical diagnosis need be a lifetime sentence of poor health. Unfortunately, finding the information on how to enjoy optimal health and well-being has not been easy for women. Any woman who is faced with the need to handle significant female-related problems finds an almost total lack of available information. In addition, books on topics for which information is available, such as premenstrual syndrome and menopause, have primarily discussed the symptoms of the problems and the standard medical treatments. These books offer little in-depth information on what women can do on their own to maintain their health and well-being.

The program in this book is set up so that you can develop your own treatment plan. All the methods you need are contained in this book. They include information on diet and nutrition, as well as a great deal of information on vitamins, minerals, and herbs for menstrual cramps and low back pain. Nutritional supplementation is a very important part of an optimal health program for women with these health-care problems. I have included programs on stress reduction, exercise, acupressure massage, deep breathing exercises, and yoga that are specifically helpful for symptoms arising from menstrual cramps and low back pain. I have also included a chapter on drug therapies so that you can be fully informed about the most effective drug treatments.

Read through the entire book first to familiarize yourself with the material. The workbook (in Chapter 2) will help you evaluate your symptoms, and the Complete Treatment Chart for Menstrual Cramps and Low Back Pain (in Chapter 3) will tell you which treatments to use for your particular set of problems. These tools are quick and easy to use and will save you countless hours of work on your own. You can discover simply and easily what will work for you.

Try all the therapies listed under your particular symptoms and you will probably find that some make you feel better than others. On a regular basis, do those techniques that provide relief of your symptoms. Establish a regimen that works for you and use it every day. This program is practical and easy to follow. It can be used by itself or in conjunction with a medical program. And best of all, it works. The feeling of wellness that can be yours with a self help program will radiate out and touch your whole life. You will have more time and energy to enjoy your work, family, and other pleasures in life. Most of my patients tell me that their lives have been positively transformed by following these beneficial self help techniques.

Identifying the Problem

1

What Are Menstrual Cramps?

Menstrual cramps, or dysmenorrhea (as physicians call it), are one of the most common health-care problems that women suffer during their reproductive years. It has been estimated that as many as 30 to 50 percent of all women suffer from pain during their menstrual period, with the incidence being highest in younger women, from teenagers to women in their thirties.

In fact, at least 10 percent of younger women have symptoms so severe that they are unable to handle their normal range of activities. Many women have to miss days of work and important social functions because any movement or activity is too painful. For the first day or two of menstruation, only bed rest or curling up on the floor in the fetal position is tolerable until the symptoms finally pass. This often happened to me during my teens and twenties.

Besides the lower abdominal pain, cramp sufferers can also experience backache, pinching and pain sensations in their inner thighs, bloating, nausea, vomiting, diarrhea, constipation, faintness, dizziness, fatigue, and headaches. For those women who must curtail their activities because of cramps, these problems translate into billions of dollars of lost wages and productivity on the job, as well as a significant decrease in the quality of life for several days each month.

In fact, the gynecology textbook that I used during my medical training estimated that menstrual cramps caused the loss of 140 million work hours annually. It is no wonder that women with moderate to severe cramps regard their monthly period with apprehension and even dread.

Despite the many symptoms and the millions of sufferers, menstrual cramps have been traditionally considered by the medical community to be a "minor" female ailment. Doctors treated women as if the problem were "all in their heads." The problem was either ignored or else treated with powerful painkilling drugs and tranquilizers. Often these drugs had significant side effects and did nothing to alleviate or help prevent the problem on a long-term basis. Luckily, the medical community's interest in menstrual cramps has increased during the past two decades. Researchers understand much more about what causes menstrual cramps on a physiological basis. This has led to newer, much more effective drug treatments, as well as nutritional and other lifestyle-related therapies.

The Normal Menstrual Cycle

It is important to look at the normal menstrual cycle and see how it functions. This background will make it easier for you to understand why painful menstruation occurs.

First, understand why we menstruate. Menstruation refers to the shedding of the uterine lining, or endometrium. Each month the uterus prepares a thick, blood-rich cushion to nourish and house a fertilized egg. If pregnancy doesn't occur and the egg doesn't implant in the uterus, then the body doesn't need this extra buildup of the uterine lining. The uterus cleanses itself by releasing the extra blood and tissue so that a fresh buildup can occur all over again the following month, in preparation for a possible pregnancy.

The mechanism that regulates the buildup and shedding of the uterine lining is controlled by fluctuations in your hormonal levels. It begins each month when follicle-stimulating hormones

(FSH) and luteinizing hormones (LH) are released from the pituitary, a gland located at the base of the brain. Once FSH and LH are released into the bloodstream, their destination is the ovaries. The ovaries hold all the eggs a woman will ever have, in an inactive form called follicles. During each cycle, the FSH and LH from the pituitary gland cause one follicle to ripen, and normally one egg is released for possible fertilization. As part of this process, the follicles begin to produce the hormones estrogen and progesterone. Estrogen reaches its peak during the first half of the cycle as the newly released egg is maturing. Progesterone output occurs after midcycle when ovulation has occurred. Ovulation refers to the production of a mature egg cell.

Besides preparing the egg for fertilization, estrogen and progesterone stimulate the lining of the uterus. During the first two weeks following menstruation, estrogen causes the uterine lining to gradually rebuild itself. The inner mucous layer of glands of the endometrium begin to grow long, and the lining thickens through an increase in the number of blood vessels as well as the production of a mesh of fibers that interconnect throughout the lining. By midcycle, the lining of the uterus has increased three times in thickness and has a greatly increased blood supply.

After midcycle, usually around day 14, ovulation occurs; the egg is picked up by the fallopian tube and continues on to the uterus. The follicle that has produced the egg for that month (*graafian follicle*) is further stimulated after midcycle by LH and changes into a yellow body, or *corpus luteum*. It is the *corpus luteum* that secretes progesterone. Progesterone has further effects on the uterine lining. It causes a coiling of the blood vessels of the lining, which becomes swollen and tortuous and secretes a thick mucous.

If the egg is fertilized, it will implant on the uterine wall and the *corpus luteum* will continue to secrete progesterone. If no fertilization occurs, the *corpus luteum* begins to deteriorate and the progesterone levels decrease. The lining of the uterus starts to break down and menstruation begins.

Types and Causes of Menstrual Cramps

There are two types of menstrual cramps: primary dysmenorrhea, in which the pain itself is the main problem; and secondary dysmenorrhea, in which the pain is a consequence of another underlying health problem.

By far the most women suffer from the primary type of dysmenorrhea. This classification breaks down into two subtypes: primary spasmodic or congestive. Primary spasmodic dysmenorrhea is the type most commonly found in young women in their early teens to late twenties. It is more common in women who have never borne children. In fact, childbearing seems to mark the end of the primary spasmodic type of cramps in many women. It is characterized by sharp, viselike pains that are caused by a constriction and tightening of the uterine muscle. Some women also feel these sharp pains in the inner thighs and low abdominal muscles, and some additionally experience feelings of hot and cold, faintness to the point of passing out, nausea, vomiting, and bowel changes varying from constipation to diarrhea. The immediate cause of the cramping is that the uterine muscle and the blood vessels that supply the uterus are tight and contracted. Blood circulation and oxygenation to this area are diminished, so the metabolism of the uterus and pelvic muscles is decreased. Waste products of metabolism, such as carbon dioxide and lactic acid, build up, intensifying the pain and discomfort.

Primary Spasmodic Dysmenorrhea

Primary spasmodic dysmenorrhea has been linked to imbalances in the intricate hormonal system that operates throughout the menstrual cycle. First, medical researchers observed that women who don't ovulate, and consequently undergo only the estrogenic effects on the lining of the uterus, do not experience cramps. Therefore, progesterone needs to be present for menstrual cramps to occur. When cramps occur, the changes seen in the lining of the uterus are typical of those occurring during an ovulatory cycle when progesterone is present. Pain-free menses without ovulation are typically seen in women at both the beginning and end of their reproductive years, that is, in young teenagers who have just started to menstruate and in women who are transitioning into menopause. There is no evidence, however, that women with cramps actually have low levels of estrogen, or conversely, high levels of progesterone. It may be the interplay between the two hormones that influences the tension and constriction in the uterine muscle and blood vessels.

In addition to the hormones estrogen and progesterone, hormonelike chemicals called prostaglandins also affect menstrual cramps. These chemicals are found in many tissues in the body, including the uterus, gastrointestinal tract, and blood vessels. There are many different types of prostaglandins, all of which affect muscle tension. However, not all prostaglandins affect muscles in the same way. Some, such as the series-two prostaglandins (specifically the E2 and F2 Alpha), trigger powerful smooth-muscle contractions. Because of this physiological effect, an overabundance of series-two prostaglandins is strongly linked to menstrual cramps and pain. These prostaglandins have also been linked to high blood pressure because they act to narrow the diameter of blood vessels. They can also trigger irritable bowel syndrome since they cause cramping of the intestinal muscles. Not all prostaglandins, however, cause muscle contraction. Others, such as the series-one and series-three, actually promote muscle relaxation and can help relieve menstrual cramps.

Prostaglandins are derived from fatty acids in the diet. The series-two prostaglandins that trigger muscle contractions are derived from animal fat—meat, dairy products, and eggs. The beneficial muscle-relaxant series-one and series-three prostaglandins are derived from vegetable and fish sources of fatty acids. These fatty acids, called linoleic acid and linolenic acid, are found predominately in raw seeds and nuts, such as flax seed or pumpkin seed, and in certain fish, such as trout, mackerel, and salmon. Thus, how we eat can actually determine which hormonal pathway we travel, leading to either muscle tension or muscle relaxation. This is a very good example of how our food selection can determine our state of health. Like progesterone, excessive prostaglandin production is seen only during ovulatory menstrual cycles. Prostaglandin production increases during the second half of the cycle, peaking toward the end of the cycle with the onset of menstruation.

Primary Congestive Dysmenorrhea

The pain that characterizes primary congestive dysmenorrhea is different from that of spasmodic cramping. Congestive symptoms produce a dull aching in the low back and pelvic region, often accompanied by bloating, weight gain, breast tenderness, headaches, and irritability. Unlike spasmodic cramping, these symptoms don't improve with age and, in some women, can worsen with age. Some of the worst symptoms are seen in women in their thirties and forties.

Women with congestive symptoms tend to retain excessive amounts of fluid and salt. Bloat accumulates in the pelvic region as well as breasts; it can cause an uncomfortable, dull aching sensation that makes these parts of the body tender to the touch. Excessive amounts of estrogen can worsen these symptoms, since estrogen increases fluid and salt retention in the body.

An excess secretion of the pituitary hormone ACTH can also worsen congestive symptoms. ACTH stimulates the production of adrenal hormones, which are then sent to the kidneys and cause the kidneys to retain fluid. As a result, women urinate less frequently in the time leading up to menstruation. Once the menstrual period starts, this excess fluid is released. Nutritional factors also influence bloating. High-salt foods should be avoided, since they increase fluid retention.

Food allergies can also contribute to congestive symptoms. Women who are sensitive to both wheat and dairy products (two of the most allergenic foods) can have a premature increase in their congestive symptoms. I have observed this in many of my patients. Other high-stress foods include alcohol, which is toxic to the liver. The liver is responsible for the breakdown of estrogen so that it can be excreted from the body. Excessive alcohol intake can increase the levels of estrogen in the body, increasing pelvic congestion. Sugar causes constriction of blood vessels, which can worsen cramps; both sugar and alcohol should be avoided in a cramp-relief program. When I put women on a salt-free, dairy-free, and wheat-free diet, the tendency to accumulate bloat decreases, as does the dull, aching abdominal discomfort and low back pain.

Other risk factors can also contribute to both spasmodic and congestive menstrual cramps. These include the following variables:

- Use of tampons may contribute to menstrual cramping in some women. Women who find that tampon use worsens their cramps should switch to sanitary napkins.

- Use of an IUD may significantly worsen the spasmodic type of cramping, and the device may need to be removed if symptoms are too severe.

- Bladder infections can cause symptoms of dull, aching pain in the lower abdominal region. Frequent bladder infections near or during menstrual periods can be a problem for some women.

- Vaginal yeast infections can occur during menstrual periods because of changes in the vaginal pH.

- Childlessness is a risk factor for spasmodic cramping; congestive symptoms may actually be worse in women who have had several pregnancies.

- Lack of exercise and poor posture increases the tendencies toward both types of cramps, since blood circulation and oxygenation is decreased.

- Stress can worsen cramps by causing women to tense their pelvic and low back muscles unconsciously.

Secondary Dysmenorrhea

The result of underlying health problems that can cause uterine and low back pain, secondary dysmenorrhea occurs most frequently in older women, typically in their forties and early fifties. Often, periods will suddenly become painful after years of pain-free menstruation. Secondary dysmenorrhea is much less common than the primary types. Some common causes of secondary dysmenorrhea include the following conditions.

Fibroid Tumors of the Uterus. Fibroid tumors occur when the muscular tissue of the uterus grows excessively. Fibroids can grow very large in some women, enlarging the uterus to sizes seen in pregnancy. If they grow large enough to impinge on the bowel and bladder, or if their growth outstrips their blood supply, they can worsen menstrual cramps. These growths occur most often in women during their reproductive years.

Fibroid tumors are stimulated by estrogen. They may expand in size with the use of estrogen-dominated birth control pills, during pregnancy, or in women who secrete high levels of estrogen naturally. Besides causing menstrual cramps, large fibroids can put pressure on the bladder or bowels, causing urinary frequency or bowel changes. Fibroids can also cause excessive menstrual bleeding and pelvic discomfort to the point of necessitating a hysterectomy. In fact, fibroids are one of the most common reasons for the 650,000 hysterectomies performed each year in the United States. Usually such tumors shrink after menopause because of the decrease in estrogen.

Pelvic Inflammatory Disease (PID). This refers to an infection of a woman's uterus, fallopian tubes, or ovaries. This serious infection must be diagnosed and treated immediately in order to prevent scarring of the reproductive organs and infertility. Symptoms of PID include fever, chills, back pain, a puslike vaginal discharge, pain during or after sexual intercourse, and spotting. When chronic, a low-grade smoldering infection can also cause lower abdominal cramps during menstruation. If untreated, the chronic menstrual pain can necessitate a hysterectomy.

Endometriosis. In this condition, pieces of the uterine lining, or endometrium, implant and grow outside the uterus in other parts of the pelvic cavity. Implants can be found on any pelvic structure, including the fallopian tubes, ovaries, and outer wall of the uterus. They can even become embedded in the intestinal and bladder walls. These tissues, like the normal lining of the uterus, are responsive to hormonal changes and can bleed with the onset of the menstrual period. Although the bleeding from the uterine lining can leave the body vaginally through menstruation, bleeding from endometrial implants in the pelvis is retained by the body and can cause scarring and inflammation over time. Pain is the most common symptom that arises from this structural damage. Women with endometriosis suffer from pain during menstruation as well as during sexual intercourse.

Treatments for endometriosis vary depending on the woman's age, severity of symptoms, and her childbearing status. Supportive therapy often includes antiprostaglandin medication such as Motrin and Ponstel. Stronger painkilling medication may be used if symptoms are severe. Pregnancy is actually a treatment for endometriosis, since it relieves monthly menstruation. In fact, doctors have traditionally recommended that women with endometriosis consider pregnancy to alleviate the problem. Unfortunately, women with endometriosis suffer from a higher level of infertility than the general population because of the scarring and other structural damage that endometriosis creates in the reproductive tract. In some cases, physicians recommend treatments including the use of birth control pills and other hormonal therapies that inhibit normal menstruation and reverse the stimulation of the endometrial implants. These therapies can be quite effective in reversing the process, but their use requires care because of the many possible side effects that can occur. In advanced cases, endometriosis may culminate in a hysterectomy.

In summary, this chapter has given you information on the different types, causes, and symptoms of menstrual cramps. As you can see, menstrual cramps can arise from a variety of conditions. To identify your specific type of menstrual cramp pattern, go on to the next chapter. Chapter 2 contains a self-evaluation workbook that will help you pinpoint the risk factors and lifestyle habits that contribute to your symptoms.

Types of Menstrual Cramps

Primary Spasmodic Dysmenorrhea
Severe viselike pain, backache, tightening and pain sensations in the inner thighs, nausea, vomiting, diarrhea, constipation, faintness, dizziness, fatigue, headaches

Primary Congestive Dysmenorrhea
Dull aching in low back and pelvis, bloating, weight gain, breast tenderness, headaches, irritability

Secondary Dysmenorrhea
Pelvic and back pain, spotting, pain during or after sexual intercourse, fever, chills, puslike vaginal discharge, urinary frequency, bowel changes

Risk Factors for Menstrual Cramps

- Use of tampons
- Use of IUD
- Bladder infections
- Yeast infections
- Childlessness (primary spasmodic dysmenorrhea)
- Multiple pregnancies (primary congestive dysmenorrhea)
- Lack of exercise
- Poor posture
- Emotional stress

Evaluating Your Symptoms

2

The Menstrual Cramps Workbook

I have developed this workbook to help you evaluate your own symptoms as well as your risk factors that can contribute to menstrual cramps. By filling out the workbook sheets you can easily recognize your weak areas and put together your own treatment program from the chapters that follow.

First, begin to fill out the monthly calendar of menstrual cramp symptoms, starting today. If you can recall your symptoms for the past month, chart these symptoms as well. The calendar will allow you to see which types of symptoms you have, as well as evaluate their severity. This will make it easier for you to pick the specific treatments for your symptoms. Then, as you follow the program, you can keep using the monthly calendars (a year's worth have been included) to check your progress.

After you've filled out the calendar, turn to the evaluations that follow the calendar section. They will help you assess specific areas of your life to see which of your habit patterns are contributing to your menstrual cramps.

When you've completed the evaluations, you will be ready to go on to the self help chapters in this book and begin your own treatment program.

Monthly Calendar of Menstrual Cramp Symptoms

Grade your symptoms as you experience them each month.

○ None ✓ Mild ◗ Moderate ● Severe

DAY OF CYCLE	1	2	3	4	5
Spasmodic Cramping					
Viselike pelvic pain					
Low back pain					
Pain in inner thighs					
Nausea and vomiting					
Diarrhea					
Constipation					
Hot and cold					
Faintness, dizziness					
Fatigue					
Headaches					
Congestive Cramping					
Dull, aching pain in pelvic region					
Backache					
Bloating					
Weight gain					
Breast tenderness					
Headaches					
Irritability					
Secondary Cramping					
Pelvic pain					
Back pain					
Spotting					
Pain during/after intercourse					
Puslike vaginal discharge					
Fever, chills					
Urinary frequency					
Bowel changes					

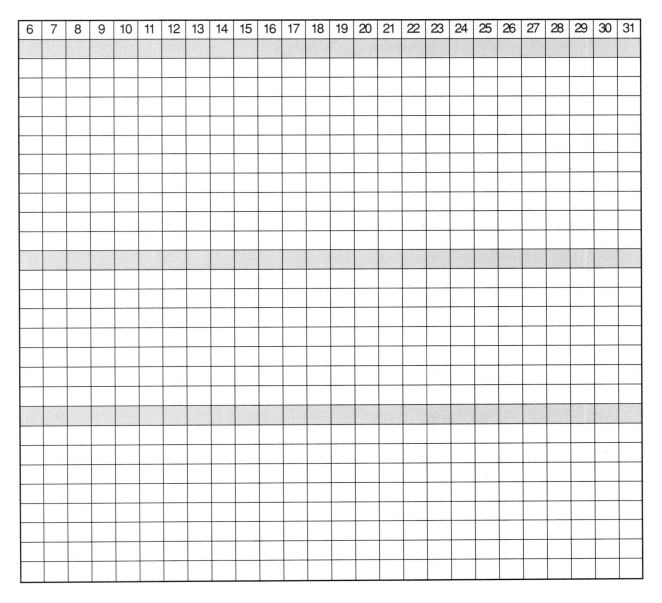

6	7	8	9	10	11	12	13	14	15	16	17	18	19	20	21	22	23	24	25	26	27	28	29	30	31

Monthly Calendar of Menstrual Cramp Symptoms

Grade your symptoms as you experience them each month.

○ None   ✓ Mild   ◗ Moderate   ● Severe

DAY OF CYCLE	1	2	3	4	5
Spasmodic Cramping					
Viselike pelvic pain					
Low back pain					
Pain in inner thighs					
Nausea and vomiting					
Diarrhea					
Constipation					
Hot and cold					
Faintness, dizziness					
Fatigue					
Headaches					
Congestive Cramping					
Dull, aching pain in pelvic region					
Backache					
Bloating					
Weight gain					
Breast tenderness					
Headaches					
Irritability					
Secondary Cramping					
Pelvic pain					
Back pain					
Spotting					
Pain during/after intercourse					
Puslike vaginal discharge					
Fever, chills					
Urinary frequency					
Bowel changes					

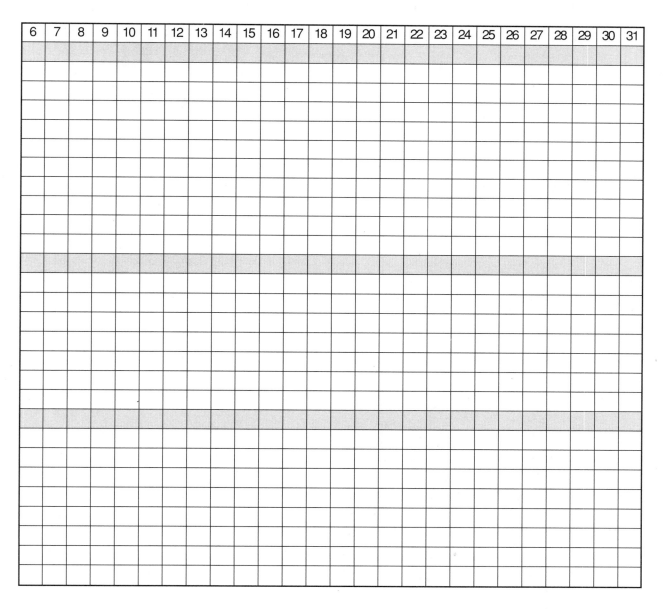

6	7	8	9	10	11	12	13	14	15	16	17	18	19	20	21	22	23	24	25	26	27	28	29	30	31

Monthly Calendar of Menstrual Cramp Symptoms

Grade your symptoms as you experience them each month.

○ None   ✓ Mild   ◗ Moderate   ● Severe

DAY OF CYCLE	1	2	3	4	5
Spasmodic Cramping					
Viselike pelvic pain					
Low back pain					
Pain in inner thighs					
Nausea and vomiting					
Diarrhea					
Constipation					
Hot and cold					
Faintness, dizziness					
Fatigue					
Headaches					
Congestive Cramping					
Dull, aching pain in pelvic region					
Backache					
Bloating					
Weight gain					
Breast tenderness					
Headaches					
Irritability					
Secondary Cramping					
Pelvic pain					
Back pain					
Spotting					
Pain during/after intercourse					
Puslike vaginal discharge					
Fever, chills					
Urinary frequency					
Bowel changes					

Month 3

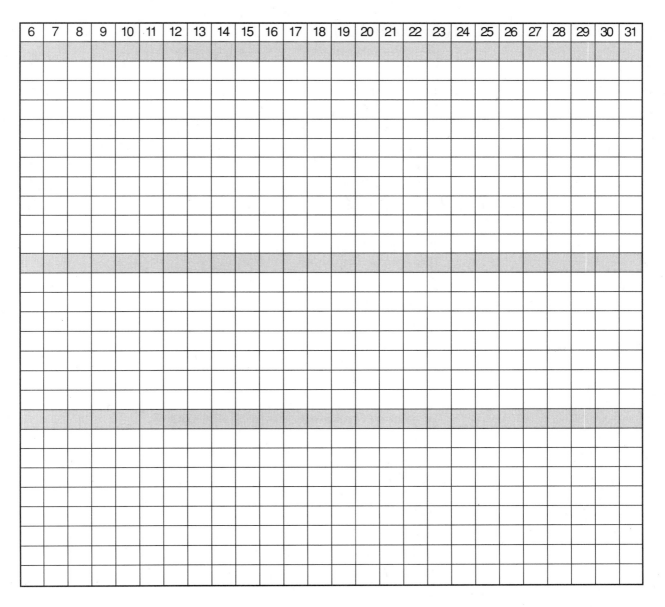

6	7	8	9	10	11	12	13	14	15	16	17	18	19	20	21	22	23	24	25	26	27	28	29	30	31

Monthly Calendar of Menstrual Cramp Symptoms

Grade your symptoms as you experience them each month.

○ None   ✓ Mild   ◗ Moderate   ● Severe

DAY OF CYCLE	1	2	3	4	5
Spasmodic Cramping					
Viselike pelvic pain					
Low back pain					
Pain in inner thighs					
Nausea and vomiting					
Diarrhea					
Constipation					
Hot and cold					
Faintness, dizziness					
Fatigue					
Headaches					
Congestive Cramping					
Dull, aching pain in pelvic region					
Backache					
Bloating					
Weight gain					
Breast tenderness					
Headaches					
Irritability					
Secondary Cramping					
Pelvic pain					
Back pain					
Spotting					
Pain during/after intercourse					
Puslike vaginal discharge					
Fever, chills					
Urinary frequency					
Bowel changes					

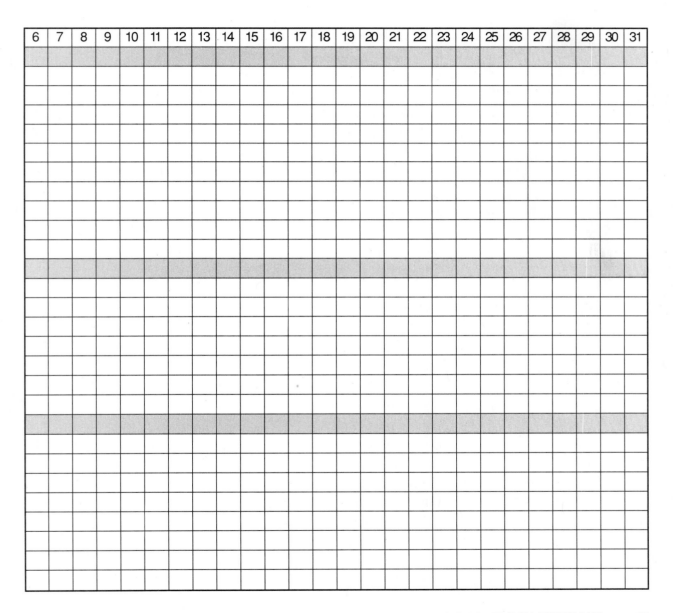

6	7	8	9	10	11	12	13	14	15	16	17	18	19	20	21	22	23	24	25	26	27	28	29	30	31

Monthly Calendar of Menstrual Cramp Symptoms

Grade your symptoms as you experience them each month.

○ None ✓ Mild ◗ Moderate ● Severe

DAY OF CYCLE	1	2	3	4	5
Spasmodic Cramping					
Viselike pelvic pain					
Low back pain					
Pain in inner thighs					
Nausea and vomiting					
Diarrhea					
Constipation					
Hot and cold					
Faintness, dizziness					
Fatigue					
Headaches					
Congestive Cramping					
Dull, aching pain in pelvic region					
Backache					
Bloating					
Weight gain					
Breast tenderness					
Headaches					
Irritability					
Secondary Cramping					
Pelvic pain					
Back pain					
Spotting					
Pain during/after intercourse					
Puslike vaginal discharge					
Fever, chills					
Urinary frequency					
Bowel changes					

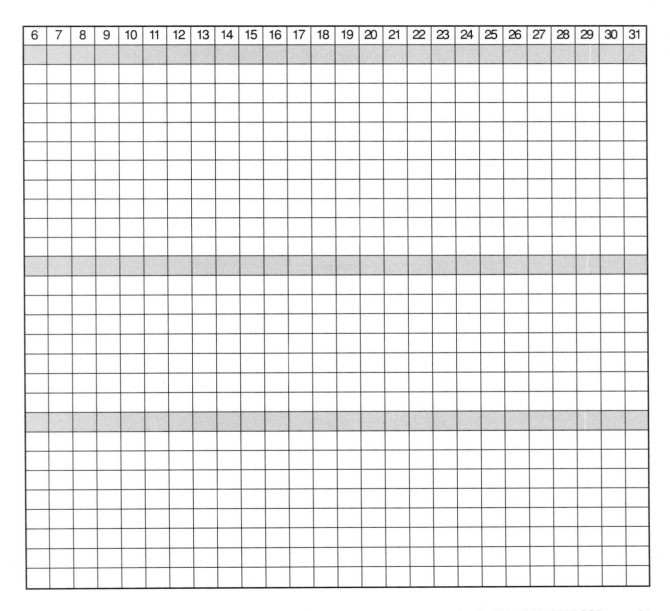

6	7	8	9	10	11	12	13	14	15	16	17	18	19	20	21	22	23	24	25	26	27	28	29	30	31

Monthly Calendar of Menstrual Cramp Symptoms

Grade your symptoms as you experience them each month.

○ None　　✓ Mild　　◗ Moderate　　● Severe

DAY OF CYCLE	1	2	3	4	5
Spasmodic Cramping					
Viselike pelvic pain					
Low back pain					
Pain in inner thighs					
Nausea and vomiting					
Diarrhea					
Constipation					
Hot and cold					
Faintness, dizziness					
Fatigue					
Headaches					
Congestive Cramping					
Dull, aching pain in pelvic region					
Backache					
Bloating					
Weight gain					
Breast tenderness					
Headaches					
Irritability					
Secondary Cramping					
Pelvic pain					
Back pain					
Spotting					
Pain during/after intercourse					
Puslike vaginal discharge					
Fever, chills					
Urinary frequency					
Bowel changes					

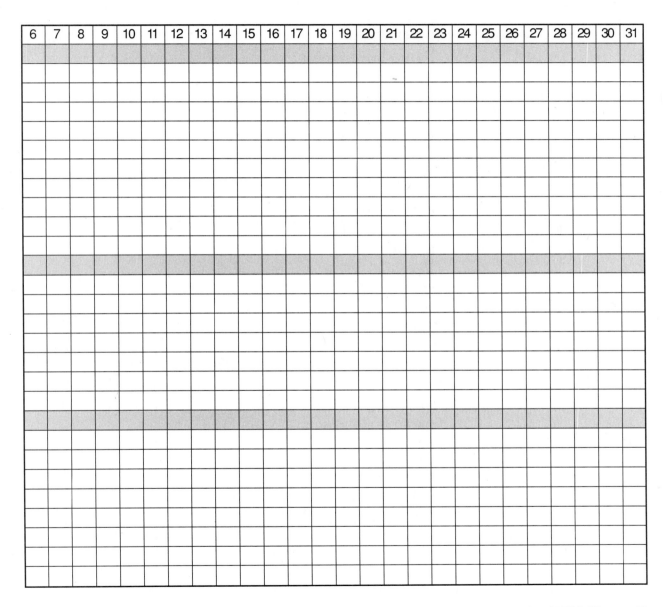

6	7	8	9	10	11	12	13	14	15	16	17	18	19	20	21	22	23	24	25	26	27	28	29	30	31

Monthly Calendar of Menstrual Cramp Symptoms

Grade your symptoms as you experience them each month.

○ None   ✓ Mild   ◗ Moderate   ● Severe

DAY OF CYCLE	1	2	3	4	5
Spasmodic Cramping					
Viselike pelvic pain					
Low back pain					
Pain in inner thighs					
Nausea and vomiting					
Diarrhea					
Constipation					
Hot and cold					
Faintness, dizziness					
Fatigue					
Headaches					
Congestive Cramping					
Dull, aching pain in pelvic region					
Backache					
Bloating					
Weight gain					
Breast tenderness					
Headaches					
Irritability					
Secondary Cramping					
Pelvic pain					
Back pain					
Spotting					
Pain during/after intercourse					
Puslike vaginal discharge					
Fever, chills					
Urinary frequency					
Bowel changes					

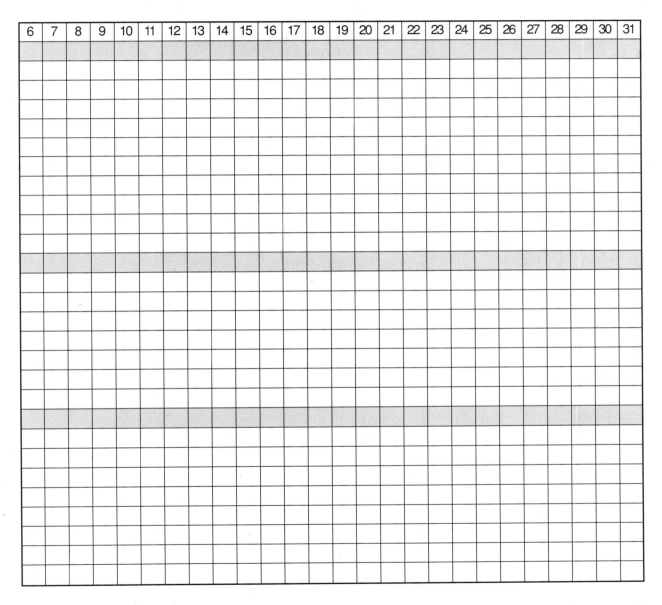

6	7	8	9	10	11	12	13	14	15	16	17	18	19	20	21	22	23	24	25	26	27	28	29	30	31

Monthly Calendar of Menstrual Cramp Symptoms

Grade your symptoms as you experience them each month.
○ None ✓ Mild ◗ Moderate ● Severe

DAY OF CYCLE	1	2	3	4	5
Spasmodic Cramping					
Viselike pelvic pain					
Low back pain					
Pain in inner thighs					
Nausea and vomiting					
Diarrhea					
Constipation					
Hot and cold					
Faintness, dizziness					
Fatigue					
Headaches					
Congestive Cramping					
Dull, aching pain in pelvic region					
Backache					
Bloating					
Weight gain					
Breast tenderness					
Headaches					
Irritability					
Secondary Cramping					
Pelvic pain					
Back pain					
Spotting					
Pain during/after intercourse					
Puslike vaginal discharge					
Fever, chills					
Urinary frequency					
Bowel changes					

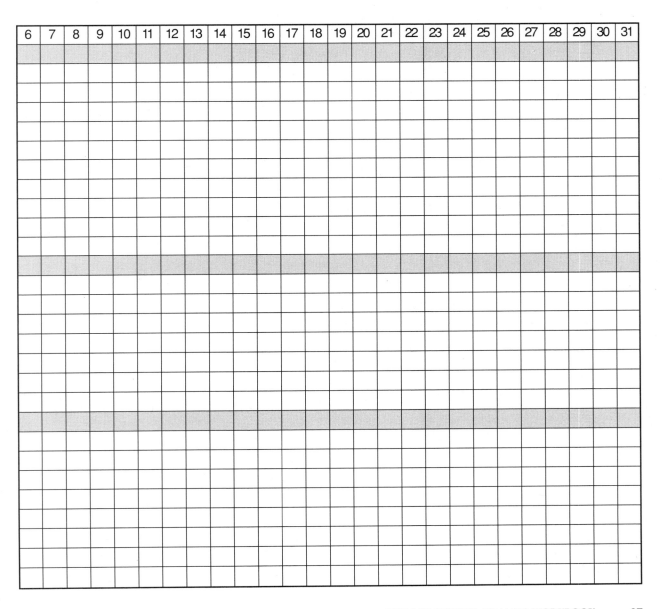

6	7	8	9	10	11	12	13	14	15	16	17	18	19	20	21	22	23	24	25	26	27	28	29	30	31

Monthly Calendar of Menstrual Cramp Symptoms

Grade your symptoms as you experience them each month.

○ None ✓ Mild ◗ Moderate ● Severe

DAY OF CYCLE	1	2	3	4	5
Spasmodic Cramping					
Viselike pelvic pain					
Low back pain					
Pain in inner thighs					
Nausea and vomiting					
Diarrhea					
Constipation					
Hot and cold					
Faintness, dizziness					
Fatigue					
Headaches					
Congestive Cramping					
Dull, aching pain in pelvic region					
Backache					
Bloating					
Weight gain					
Breast tenderness					
Headaches					
Irritability					
Secondary Cramping					
Pelvic pain					
Back pain					
Spotting					
Pain during/after intercourse					
Puslike vaginal discharge					
Fever, chills					
Urinary frequency					
Bowel changes					

6	7	8	9	10	11	12	13	14	15	16	17	18	19	20	21	22	23	24	25	26	27	28	29	30	31

Monthly Calendar of Menstrual Cramp Symptoms

Grade your symptoms as you experience them each month.

○ None   ✓ Mild   ◗ Moderate   ● Severe

DAY OF CYCLE	1	2	3	4	5
Spasmodic Cramping					
Viselike pelvic pain					
Low back pain					
Pain in inner thighs					
Nausea and vomiting					
Diarrhea					
Constipation					
Hot and cold					
Faintness, dizziness					
Fatigue					
Headaches					
Congestive Cramping					
Dull, aching pain in pelvic region					
Backache					
Bloating					
Weight gain					
Breast tenderness					
Headaches					
Irritability					
Secondary Cramping					
Pelvic pain					
Back pain					
Spotting					
Pain during/after intercourse					
Puslike vaginal discharge					
Fever, chills					
Urinary frequency					
Bowel changes					

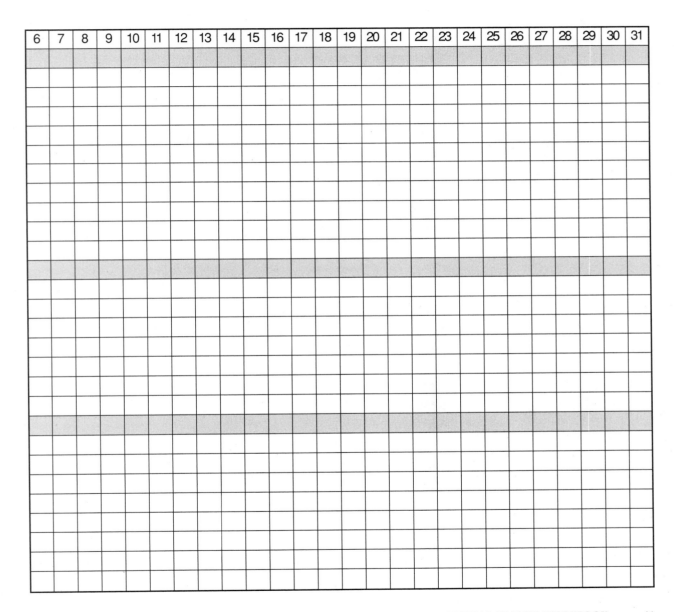

6	7	8	9	10	11	12	13	14	15	16	17	18	19	20	21	22	23	24	25	26	27	28	29	30	31

Monthly Calendar of Menstrual Cramp Symptoms

Grade your symptoms as you experience them each month.

○ None ✓ Mild ◗ Moderate ● Severe

DAY OF CYCLE	1	2	3	4	5
Spasmodic Cramping					
Viselike pelvic pain					
Low back pain					
Pain in inner thighs					
Nausea and vomiting					
Diarrhea					
Constipation					
Hot and cold					
Faintness, dizziness					
Fatigue					
Headaches					
Congestive Cramping					
Dull, aching pain in pelvic region					
Backache					
Bloating					
Weight gain					
Breast tenderness					
Headaches					
Irritability					
Secondary Cramping					
Pelvic pain					
Back pain					
Spotting					
Pain during/after intercourse					
Puslike vaginal discharge					
Fever, chills					
Urinary frequency					
Bowel changes					

6	7	8	9	10	11	12	13	14	15	16	17	18	19	20	21	22	23	24	25	26	27	28	29	30	31

Monthly Calendar of Menstrual Cramp Symptoms

Grade your symptoms as you experience them each month.

○ None　　✓ Mild　　◗ Moderate　　● Severe

DAY OF CYCLE	1	2	3	4	5
Spasmodic Cramping					
Viselike pelvic pain					
Low back pain					
Pain in inner thighs					
Nausea and vomiting					
Diarrhea					
Constipation					
Hot and cold					
Faintness, dizziness					
Fatigue					
Headaches					
Congestive Cramping					
Dull, aching pain in pelvic region					
Backache					
Bloating					
Weight gain					
Breast tenderness					
Headaches					
Irritability					
Secondary Cramping					
Pelvic pain					
Back pain					
Spotting					
Pain during/after intercourse					
Puslike vaginal discharge					
Fever, chills					
Urinary frequency					
Bowel changes					

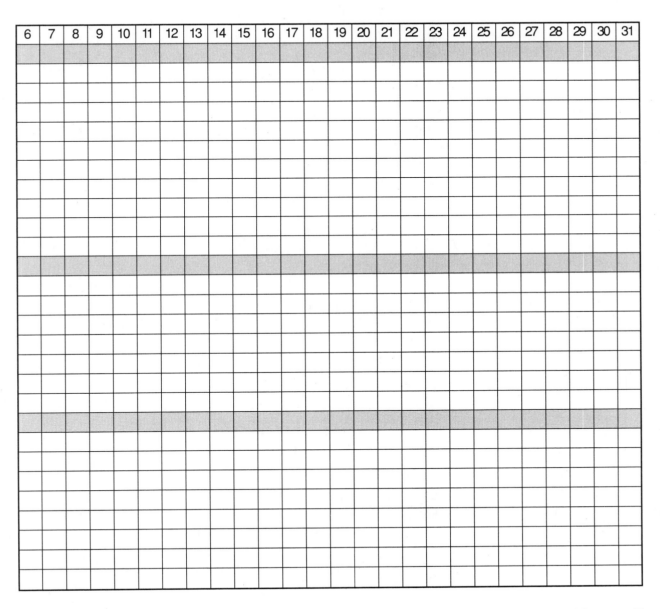

6	7	8	9	10	11	12	13	14	15	16	17	18	19	20	21	22	23	24	25	26	27	28	29	30	31

Risk Factors for Menstrual Cramps

You are at higher risk of menstrual cramps if you have any of the risk factors listed below. Be sure to follow the nutritional, exercise, and stress-management guidelines in the self-help section of this book if you have any of the related risk factors for menstrual cramps listed here. Check each risk factor that applies to you.

Risk Factors

Use of tampons	___
Use of IUD	___
Recurrent bladder infections	___
Recurrent yeast infections	___
Childlessness (spasmodic cramps)	___
Multiple pregnancies (congestive cramps)	___
Endometriosis	___
Fibroid tumors	___
Pelvic inflammatory disease (PID)	___
Lack of exercise	___
Poor posture	___
Emotional stress	___
Daily use of: Salt	___
Animal fats	___
Dairy products	___
Wheat	___
Alcohol	___
Sugar	___

Eating Habits and Menstrual Cramps

All foods in the shaded area of the following checklist are high-stress foods that can worsen menstrual cramps. If you eat a substantial number of these foods, or if you eat any of these foods frequently, your nutritional habits may be contributing significantly to your symptoms. Read the chapters on beneficial foods, meal plans, and recipes for further guidance on food selection.

All the foods from avocado to fish are high-nutrient, low-stress foods that may help to relieve or prevent menstrual cramp symptoms. These foods should be included frequently in your diet. If you are already eating many of these foods and few of the high-stress foods, chances are your nutritional habits are good, and food selection may not be a significant factor in worsening your menstrual cramps. You may want to look carefully at the stress management and exercise chapters. The activities contained in these chapters may be very helpful in relieving your cramps.

Eating Habit Checklist

Check the number of times you eat the following foods:

Foods	Never	Once a Month	Once a Week	Twice a Week +
Cow's milk				
Cow's cheese				
Butter				
Yogurt				
Eggs				
Chocolate				
Sugar				
Alcohol				
Beef				
Pork				
Lamb				
Wheat bread				
Wheat noodles				
Wheat-based flour				
Pastries				
Added salt				
Bouillon				
Commercial salad dressing				
Catsup				

Foods	Never	Once a Month	Once a Week	Twice a Week +
Coffee				
Black tea				
Soft drinks				
Hot dogs				
Ham				
Bacon				
Avocado				
Beans				
Beets				
Broccoli				
Brussels sprouts				
Cabbage				
Carrots				
Celery				
Collards				
Cucumbers				
Eggplant				
Garlic				
Horseradish				
Kale				
Lettuce				
Mustard greens				
Okra				
Onions				
Parsnips				
Peas				
Potatoes				
Radishes				
Rutabagas				
Spinach				
Squash				
Sweet potatoes				

Foods	Never	Once a Month	Once a Week	Twice a Week +
Tomatoes				
Turnips				
Turnip greens				
Yams				
Brown rice				
Millet				
Barley				
Oatmeal				
Buckwheat				
Rye				
Raw flax seeds				
Corn				
Raw pumpkin seeds				
Raw sesame seeds				
Raw sunflower seeds				
Raw almonds				
Raw filberts				
Raw pecans				
Raw walnuts				
Apples				
Bananas				
Berries				
Pears				
Seasonal fruits				
Corn oil				
Flax oil				
Olive oil				
Sesame oil				
Safflower oil				
Poultry				
Fish				

Exercise Habits and Menstrual Cramps

Exercise helps prevent menstrual cramps by relaxing muscles and promoting better blood circulation and oxygenation to the pelvic area. It can also help reduce stress and relieve anxiety and upset. If your total number of exercise periods per week is less than three, you will probably be more prone to cramp symptoms. See the chapters on the various kinds of exercise that can help relieve and prevent symptoms.

If you are exercising more than three times a week, keep doing your exercises; they are probably making your symptoms less severe. You may want to add specific corrective exercises to your present regimen, choosing them to fit your individual symptoms. There are many options available in the chapters on exercise, yoga, and acupressure massage.

Exercise Checklist

Check the frequency with which you do any of the following:

Exercise	Never	Once a Month	Once a Week	Twice a Week +
Walking				
Running				
Dancing				
Swimming				
Bicycling				
Tennis				
Stretching				
Yoga				

Stress Evaluation Tool

If you are experiencing any of the following life events, check those that apply to you.

Checking many items in the first third of this scale indicates major life stress and a possible vulnerability to serious illness. In other words, the more items checked in the first two thirds, the higher your stress quotient. *Do everything possible to manage your stress in a healthy way.* Eat the foods that provide a high-nutrient/low-stress diet, exercise on a regular basis, and learn the methods for managing stress given in the chapter on stress reduction and deep breathing.

If you check fewer items, you are probably at lower risk for illness. Because stresses too minimal to include in this evaluation may also play a part in increasing your menstrual cramps, you will still benefit from practicing the methods outlined in the chapter on stress reduction. Stress management is very important in helping you to gain control over your level of muscle tension.

Check if this stressful event applies to you.

Life Events

____ Death of spouse or close family member

____ Divorce from spouse

____ Death of a close friend

____ Legal separation from spouse

____ Loss of job

____ Radical loss of financial security

____ Major personal injury or illness (gynecologic or other cause)

____ Future surgery for gynecologic or other illness

____ Beginning a new marriage

____ Foreclosure of mortgage or loan

____ Lawsuit lodged against you

_____ Marriage reconciliation

_____ Change in health of a family member

_____ Major trouble with boss or co-workers

_____ Increase in responsibility—job or home

_____ Learn you are pregnant

_____ Difficulties with your sexual abilities

_____ Gaining a new family member

_____ Change to a different job

_____ Increase in number of marital arguments

_____ New loan or mortgage of more than $100,000

_____ Son or daughter leaving home

_____ Major disagreement with in-laws or friends

_____ Spouse begins or stops work

_____ Recognition for outstanding achievements

_____ Begin or end education

_____ Undergo a change in living conditions

_____ Revise or alter your personal habits

_____ Change in work hours or conditions

_____ Change of residence

_____ Change your school or major in school

_____ Alterations in your recreation activities

_____ Change in church or club activities

_____ Change in social activities

_____ Change in sleeping habits

_____ Change in number of family get-togethers

_____ Diet or eating habits are changed

_____ You go on vacation

_____ The year-end holidays occur

_____ You commit a minor violation of the law

Major life stress can have a significant impact on the symptoms of menstrual cramps as well as other health problems. It is helpful to assess your own level of stress to see how it may be impacting your health. One popular tool is the Holmes and Rahe Social Readjustment Rating Scale, first published in 1967. The scale above is adapted for women and identifies events that cause stress.

Daily Stress Evaluation

This evaluation is a very important one for women with a tendency toward menstrual cramps. Not all stresses have a major impact on our lives, as do death, divorce, or personal injury. Most of us are exposed to a multitude of small life stresses on a daily basis. The effects of these stresses are cumulative and can be a major factor in triggering muscle tension in the pelvic area on an unconscious basis.

Check each item that seems to apply to you.

Work

_____ **Too much responsibility.** You feel you have to push too hard to do your work. There are too many demands made of you. You feel very pressured by all of this responsibility. You worry about getting all your work done and doing it well.

_____ **Time urgency.** You worry about getting your work done on time. You always feel rushed. It feels like there are not enough hours in the day to complete your work.

_____ **Job instability.** You are concerned about losing your job. There are layoffs at your company. There is much insecurity and concern among your fellow employees about their job security.

____ **Job performance.** You don't feel that you are working up to your maximum capability because of outside pressures or stress. You are unhappy with your own job performance and concerned about job security as a result.

____ **Difficulty getting along with co-workers and boss.** Your boss is too picky and critical. Your boss demands too much. You must work closely with co-workers who are difficult to get along with.

____ **Understimulation.** Work is boring. The lack of stimulation makes you tired. You wish you were somewhere else.

____ **Uncomfortable physical plant.** Lights are too bright or too dim; noises are too loud. You're exposed to noxious fumes or chemicals. There is too much activity going on around you, making it difficult to concentrate.

Spouse or Significant Other

____ **Hostile communication.** There is too much negative emotion and drama. You are always upset and angry. There is not enough peace and quiet.

____ **Not enough communication.** There is not enough discussion of feelings or issues. You both tend to hold in your feelings. You feel that an emotional bond is lacking between you.

____ **Discrepancy in communication.** One person talks about feelings too much, the other person too little.

____ **Affection.** You do not feel you receive enough affection. There is not enough holding, touching, and loving in your relationship. Or, you are made uncomfortable by your partner's demands for affection.

____ **Sexuality.** There is not enough sexual intimacy. You feel deprived by your partner. Or, there is a demand for too-frequent sexual relations by your partner. You feel pressured.

____ **Children.** They make too much noise. They make too many demands on your time. They are hard to discipline.

____ **Organization.** Home is poorly organized. It always seems messy; chores are half-finished.

____ **Time.** There is too much to do in the home and never enough time to get it all done.

____ **Responsibility.** You need more help. There are too many demands on your time and energy.

Your Emotional State

____ **Too much anxiety.** You worry too much about every little thing. You constantly worry about what can go wrong in your life.

____ **Victimization.** Everyone is taking advantage of you or wants to hurt you.

____ **Poor self-image.** You don't like yourself enough. You are always finding fault with yourself.

____ **Too critical.** You are always finding fault with others. You always look at what is wrong with other people rather than seeing their virtues.

_____ **Inability to relax.** You are always wound up. It is difficult for you to relax. You are tense and restless.

_____ **Not enough self-renewal.** You don't play enough or take enough time off to relax and have fun. As a result, life isn't fun and enjoyable.

_____ **Too angry.** Small life issues seem to upset you unduly. You find yourself becoming angry and irritable with your husband, children, or clients.

Read over the day-to-day stress areas that you find difficult to handle. How many items have you checked? Becoming aware of them is the first step toward lessening their effects on your life. Methods for reducing them and helping your body to deal with them are given in the chapter on stress reduction.

How Stress Affects Your Body

This evaluation should help you become aware of where stress localizes in your body. Each woman accumulates stress in a different way, tensing and contracting different sets of muscles in a pattern that is unique to her. This accumulation increases your level of fatigue and lowers your energy and vitality. Storing tension in the low back and pelvic area can worsen cramps, while storing it in the neck can cause headaches.

Check the places where tension most commonly localizes in your body.

_____ Low back
_____ Pelvic area
_____ Stomach muscles
_____ Thighs and calves
_____ Chest
_____ Shoulders
_____ Arms
_____ Neck and throat
_____ Headache
_____ Grinding teeth
_____ Eyestrain

It is important to be aware of where you store tension in the body. When you feel tension building up in these areas, begin deep breathing or use one of the other methods given in the chapter on stress reduction. Often, these techniques will help to release muscle tension rapidly.

Finding
the Solution

3

The Menstrual Cramps Self Help Program— Complete Treatment Chart

The preceding section has given you much useful information about symptoms and causes of menstrual cramps and low back pain. You are now ready to put together your own self help treatment program. I have included in this part of the book many treatment methods that I have found to be very helpful with my own patients. These treatment options include dietary and nutritional supplement programs as well as programs for stress management, exercise, breathing exercises, acupressure massage, and yoga. Each section presents specific information and techniques to help relieve and prevent your symptoms.

The program is set up so that you can individualize a treatment plan for yourself. This chapter contains a summary chart that will help you put your own program together.

You can use the summary chart in two ways. First, when you begin your program, I recommend that you try all the therapies that pique your interest. You will probably find that some therapies make you feel better than others. Establish the regimen that works for you and practice it on a regular basis. Alternatively, you can read straight through the rest of the book to get a general overview of the various treatment techniques. Find the treatments you are interested in trying. You can then use the treatment chart for an overview and for quick spot work.

Either way of working with the book can bring you tremendous benefits. The most important thing is to follow your program on a regular basis. This will enable you to see improvement in your health and vitality very quickly—many women begin to feel better within a month or two.

Complete Treatment Chart for Menstrual Cramps and Low Back Pain

Nutrition	Menstrual cramps dietary principles and recipes in Chapters 4 and 5. Avoid dairy products, eggs, red meat, chocolate, coffee, soft drinks, alcohol, salt, sugar
Vitamins and Minerals	Menstrual cramp formula with emphasis on vitamin B_3, vitamin B_6, vitamin C, calcium, magnesium, potassium, zinc, essential fatty acids
Herbs	ginger, ginkgo biloba, white willow bark, red raspberry leaf, cramp bark, chamomile, hops, chaste tree berry
Medication	aspirin, Advil, Midol, Pamprin, Nuprin, Naprosyn, Anaprox, Ponstel, Motrin, Tylenol with codeine, Darvon, Valium, birth control pills, Danazol, Lupron
Breathing Exercises	Breathing exercises 1, 2, 3, 4, 5, 6, 7
Stress Reduction	Stress Reduction exercises 1, 2, 3, 4, 5, 6, 7
Physical Exercise	Exercise routines 1, 2, 3, 4, 5, 6
Acupressure Massage	Acupressure massage 1, 2, 3, 4, 5
Yoga	Rock and Roll, Pelvic Arch, Cat Cow, Pump, Locust, Bow, Child's Pose, Wide-Angle Pose, Sponge

4

Dietary Principles for Menstrual Cramps

A healthy diet is the cornerstone of a good menstrual cramp self-care program. In fact, I have found that good nutritional habits bring more relief from cramps than any other single factor. Even women who have severe cramps and have used many strong drugs to suppress their symptoms benefit greatly from a proper anticramp diet. I have been very impressed by how many women have reported a noticeable decrease in their pain and discomfort within one or two menstrual cycles after starting my program. Besides the specific benefits these dietary principles will have on your cramps, they will also aid your general health and well-being. Many women have reported that they have more energy and a greater sense of well-being than they have had in years. Often they tell me that symptoms they never associated with their menstrual cramps, such as allergies and general poor digestive function, have cleared up, too.

In this chapter, I discuss in detail which foods worsen menstrual cramps and should be avoided. This list may surprise you, because it contains not only foods that are stressful to the body and are often called "junk foods," but also many foods that are staples of the American diet. Many women eat a diet that they mistakenly think is healthy, not realizing that their food selection is actually contributing to their cramps. Luckily, the list of foods that help to relieve and prevent menstrual cramps is a long one.

Once you shift to a diet of more healthful foods, you will find that they are just as delicious, convenient, and easy to prepare as the foods you are eating now. The information on these foods is the result of almost two decades of work with women who came to me with menstrual cramps and had significant relief of their symptoms. I hope you will experience the same great results.

Foods That Help Treat or Prevent Menstrual Cramps

You should emphasize in your diet the foods listed in this section. They provide the range of nutrients you need to prevent menstrual cramps and the many associated symptoms that can occur several days each month. Although your symptoms are limited to the days preceding menstruation and its onset, these foods should form the mainstay of your diet throughout the entire month. A poorly chosen high-stress diet during your symptom-free time will increase the severity of your symptoms when menstruation starts.

Whole Grains. I strongly recommend the use of whole grains such as millet, oats, and rice. Many women also tolerate 100 percent rye. These grains are excellent sources of magnesium, which helps reduce neuromuscular tension and thereby decrease menstrual cramps. They are also fairly high in calcium, which also relaxes muscle contraction. They are excellent sources of potassium, as is buckwheat. Potassium has a diuretic effect on the body tissues and helps reduce bloating. Excessive fluid retention is one of the main causes of the congestive symptoms seen with cramps, characterized by dull, aching pain.

Women with cramps should avoid eating wheat. This probably comes as a surprise to you because wheat is a mainstay of the American diet. However, wheat contains a protein called gluten that is difficult to digest and can be highly allergenic. In many of my patients with cramps, wheat has worsened symptoms such as fatigue, depression, bloating, constipation, diarrhea, and intestinal cramps. You may want to try a wheat-free diet to see if you feel better after wheat is eliminated. If you have more severe gluten intolerance or food allergies, you may want to eliminate oat and rye also, since they also contain some gluten. You may find that you feel best using buckwheat, corn, and rice. Even these grains should be rotated and used only every few days by women who have food allergies and menstrual cramps.

Another benefit of whole grains is their fiber or bran content. Bran can help reduce the congestive symptoms of cramps since it produces bulkier stools with a higher water content; this helps to get rid of excess fluid in the body. Fiber is also helpful in eliminating the digestive symptoms that occur with cramps. It has a normalizing effect on the bowel movements, helping prevent both constipation and diarrhea. Besides removing excessive water from the body, whole grains appear to help bind fat and remove it from the body, as well as helping lower cholesterol. Oat and rice bran are particularly good for this purpose. Because cancer of the breast, uterus, ovaries, and colon are linked to a diet high in animal fats, the use of whole grains may actually have a protective effect in preventing the development of these diseases.

Whole grains have other benefits, too. They are an excellent source of B-complex vitamins and vitamin E. These nutrients can help combat the fatigue and depressive symptoms seen with the onset of menstruation. They are also an excellent source of protein, particularly when combined with beans and peas.

Whole Grain Cereals. Puffed millet, unsweetened granola, puffed corn, and puffed rice are all available as cold breakfast cereals. Cream of rye, buckwheat groats, brown rice, millet, and oatmeal are excellent hot cereals. These are low-stress cereals because they are gluten-free. These products can be found easily in health food stores. Health food stores offer a wide choice of cereals rich in minerals and fiber. Your best bet if you shop in a local supermarket is the slow-cooking oatmeal (the quick-cooking kind is a refined grain product and should be avoided).

Whole Grain Breads. Health food stores offer many different gluten-free whole grain breads including those made of rice, rye, sesame-millet, soy-potato, and lima beans. Choose brands made without added sugar.

Crackers. Both rye and rice crackers are available in grocery stores. Rye flour, in particular, is a good source of potassium. Crackers can be used for snacks or open-face sandwiches. Brown rice cakes are particularly good served with soy spreads, tuna salad, or fruit and nut spreads.

Pancakes. You can make pancakes with buckwheat, rice flour, or triticale. Concentrated sweeteners such as maple syrup, honey, and applesauce can be used in small amounts.

Pasta. Pasta made of buckwheat, rice, corn, or soy is readily available in health food and ethnic food stores. These types of pasta are easy to digest for women who get digestive symptoms and bloating with menstruation.

Legumes. Beans and peas are excellent sources of calcium, magnesium, and potassium. I highly recommend their use in an anti-cramp diet. Particularly good sources of these nutrients include tofu, black beans, pinto beans, kidney beans, chickpeas, lentils, lima beans, and soybeans. These foods are also high in iron and tend to be good sources of copper and zinc. Legumes are very high in B-complex vitamins and vitamin B6, all necessary nutrients for the relief and prevention of cramps and menstrual fatigue. They are also excellent sources of protein and provide all the essential amino acids when eaten with grains. (Good examples of grain and legume combinations include meals such as beans and rice, or corn bread and split pea soup.) Legumes provide an excellent and easily utilized source of protein and can be used as a substitute for meat.

As with grains, legumes are an excellent source of fiber and can help normalize bowel function. They digest slowly and can help to regulate the blood sugar level, a trait they share with whole grains. As a result, they are an excellent food for women with diabetes or blood sugar imbalances. Some women find that gas is a problem when they eat beans. You can minimize this by using digestive enzymes, such as hydrochloric acid, and eating beans in small quantities.

Vegetables. These are outstanding foods for all menstrual cramp symptoms. Many vegetables are high in calcium, magnesium, and potassium, which help relieve and prevent the spasmodic symptoms of cramps. Besides helping to relax tense, irritable muscles, these minerals also calm and relax emotions. Both calcium and magnesium act as natural tranquilizers, a real benefit for women suffering from menstrual pain, discomfort, and irritability. Potassium aids in relieving the symptoms of congestive dysmenorrhea by reducing fluid retention and bloating. Some of the best sources for these minerals include Swiss chard, spinach, broccoli, beet greens, mustard greens, sweet potatoes, kale, potatoes, peas, and green beans. These vegetables are also high in iron, which may help to reduce cramps.

Many vegetables are high in vitamin C, which helps to increase capillary permeability and facilitate the flow of essential nutrients into the tight muscles as well as the flow of waste products out. Vitamin C is an important antistress vitamin because it is needed for healthy adrenal hormonal production (the adrenals are glands that help us deal with stress). Vitamin C is also important for immune function and wound healing. Its anti-infectious properties may help to reduce the tendency toward bladder and vaginal infections, which can cause secondary dysmenorrhea. Vegetables high in vitamin C include brussels sprouts, broccoli, cauliflower, kale, peppers, parsley, peas, tomatoes, and potatoes.

Fruits. Fruits contain a wide range of nutrients that can benefit menstrual cramps. Like many vegetables, fruits are an excellent source of vitamin C, which is important for healthy blood vessels and blood circulation into the tense pelvic muscles. Almost all fruits contain some vitamin C, with the best sources including berries, oranges, grapefruits, and melons. These fruits are also good sources of bioflavonoids, another essential nutrient that affects blood vessel strength and permeability.

Certain fruits are also excellent sources of calcium and magnesium; you can eat them often for your mineral needs. These include dried figs, raisins, blackberries, bananas, and oranges. Figs, raisins, and bananas are also exceptional sources of potassium, so should be eaten by women with fatigue and bloating. All fruits, in fact, are an excellent source of potassium.

Eat fruits whole to take advantage of their high fiber content. This fiber content helps prevent constipation and the other digestive irregularities frequently seen with menstrual cramps.

Fresh and dried fruits are excellent snack and dessert substitutes for cookies, candies, cakes, and other foods high in refined sugar. Although fruit is high in sugar, its high fiber content helps to slow down absorption of the sugar into the blood circulation and thereby helps to stabilize the blood sugar level. I recommend, however, using fruit juices in small quantities. Fruit juice does not contain the bulk or fiber of the whole fruit. As a result, it acts more like table sugar and can destabilize your blood sugar level in a dramatic manner when used to excess. In this case, less is better. If you want to have fruit juice on a more frequent basis, mix it half-and-half with water.

Seeds and Nuts. Seeds and nuts are the best sources of the two essential fatty acids, linoleic acid and linolenic acid. These provide the raw materials your body needs to produce the muscle-relaxant prostaglandin hormones. Adequate levels of essential fatty acids in your diet are very important in treating and preventing muscle cramps; they are also beneficial for your skin and hair. The best sources of both fatty acids are raw flax and pumpkin seeds. Other seeds, such as sesame and sunflower seeds, are excellent sources of linoleic acid alone. Seeds and nuts are excellent sources of the

B-complex vitamins and vitamin E, which are important antistress factors for women with cramps. These nutrients also help to regulate hormonal balance. Seeds and nuts are very high in other essential nutrients that women have a strong need for, including magnesium, calcium, and potassium. Particularly good to eat are sesame seeds, sunflower seeds, pistachios, pecans, and almonds. Because they are very high in calories, they should be eaten in small amounts.

The oils in seeds and nuts are very perishable, so exposure to light, heat, and oxygen should be avoided. Try to eat them raw, and remove them yourself from their protective shells. Seeds and nuts should be eaten raw and unsalted to get the benefit of their essential fatty acids and to avoid the negative effects of too much salt. If you buy them already shelled, they should be refrigerated so their oils don't become rancid. Seeds and nuts make a wonderful garnish on salads, vegetable dishes, and casseroles and can be eaten as a main source of protein with snacks and light meals.

Meat, Poultry, and Fish. I generally recommend eating meat only in small quantities or avoiding it entirely if you have cramps. This is because red meats like beef, pork, and lamb, as well as poultry, contain the saturated fats that the body uses to produce the series-two prostaglandins—the hormonelike chemicals that trigger muscle contraction and constriction in blood vessels, thereby worsening cramps. If you want to eat meat, I recommend that you eat fish. Unlike other meat, fish contains linolenic acid, one of the beneficial fatty acids that helps to relax muscles through the pathway. Fish are also excellent sources of minerals, especially iodine and potassium. Particularly good types of fish for women with menstrual cramps include salmon, tuna, mackerel, and trout.

If you do include meat in your cramp-relief program, I recommend that you use it in very small amounts (3 ounces or less per day). Most Americans eat much more protein than is healthy. Excessive amounts of protein are difficult to digest and stress the kidneys. Except for fish, meat is a main source of unhealthy saturated fats, which put you at higher risk of heart disease and cancer. Instead of using meat as your only or primary source of protein, I recommend that you increase your intake of grains, beans, and raw seeds and nuts, which contain protein as well as many other important nutrients. For many years I have recommended to my patients that they use meat more as a garnish and a flavoring for casseroles, stir-fries, and soups. I also recommend that you buy meat from organic, range-fed sources—this meat has undergone less exposure to pesticides, antibiotics, and hormones. If you find meat difficult to digest, you may be deficient in hydrochloric acid, a digestive enzyme normally found in the stomach. Try taking a small amount of hydrochloric acid with every meat-containing meal to see if your digestion improves.

Oils. You can use vegetable oils in small amounts for cooking, stir-frying, and sautéing; select oils such as soybean oil and corn oil that contain vitamin E. Vitamin E is an important nutrient in reducing the mood symptoms, fatigue, and cramps that occur at the onset of menstruation in those women whose cramps are due to fibroids. Medical studies show that vitamin E may help to regulate the estrogen/progesterone ratio. This is important because high levels of estrogen stimulate the growth of fibroid tumors. Women with fibroids should take vitamin E in both supplemental form and dietary sources such as wheat germ oil. In fact, wheat germ oil contains the highest levels of vitamin E and is the source for most natural vitamin E sold on the market today. Oils should be cold-pressed because this helps ensure freshness and purity. Keep your oils refrigerated to avoid rancidity.

Foods to Avoid with Menstrual Cramps

If you have menstrual cramps, you should avoid or use only in limited amounts the foods described in this section, because they can increase your monthly symptoms. You will also notice that some of these food are generally recognized as being high-stress, unhealthy foods for the body.

Dairy Products. Dairy products are a high-risk food for women with menstrual cramps. This is always a surprise to women, because dairy products have traditionally been touted as one of the four basic food groups, and most women use them as staples in their diet, consuming large amounts of cheese, yogurt, milk, and cottage cheese. Yet, dairy products are the main dietary source of arachidonic acid, the fat that your body uses to produce the muscle-contracting series-two prostaglandins. I have seen the severity of menstrual cramps decrease by as much as one-third to one-half within one menstrual cycle when women completely eliminate dairy products from their diet. The high saturated-fat content of dairy products is a risk factor for promoting excess estrogen levels in the body. Excessive estrogen is a trigger for fibroid tumors, a cause of secondary dysmenorrhea. Also, the high salt content of dairy products increases the bloating and fluid retention of congestive dysmenorrhea.

Dairy products have many other unhealthy effects on a woman's body. The tryptophan in milk has a sedative effect that increases fatigue, a real problem for some women the first day or two of their periods. Many people are allergic to dairy products or lack the enzymes to digest milk. The result can be digestive problems like bloating, gas, and bowel changes, which intensify with menstruation. Intolerance to dairy products can hamper the absorption and assimilation of the calcium they contain. Dairy products have also been shown in clinical studies to decrease iron absorption in anemic women.

Because dairy products are a risk factor for cramps, women who have depended on dairy products for their calcium intake naturally wonder about what alternative sources to use. Women who are concerned about their calcium intake can use the many other good dietary sources of this essential nutrient. These include beans, peas, soybeans, sesame seeds, soup stock made from chicken or fish bones, and green leafy vegetables. For food preparation, potato milk, soy milk, and nut milk are excellent substitutes. You can also use a supplement containing calcium, magnesium, and vitamin D to make sure your intake is sufficient. Nondairy milks are readily available at health food stores.

Fats. Like dairy products, the use of saturated fats (which generally come from animal sources, though also from a few vegetable sources, such as palm oil or coconut oil) can intensify menstrual cramps through stimulating the production of the muscle-contracting prostaglandins. In the typical American diet, 40 percent of the calories come from fat. Most of this fat is from unhealthy saturated sources such as dairy products, red meat, and eggs. This diet also tends to promote fibroid tumor growth and heavy menstrual flow in susceptible women, because excessive saturated fat intake is stressful to the liver and helps to increase excess estrogen levels. Fibroids can worsen cramps when they grow to be too large, cutting off their own blood supply and pressing on the bladder and intestines.

Saturated fat, primarily from animal sources, also puts women at high risk for heart disease and cancer of the breast, uterus, and ovaries. Women on a high-fat diet also tend to accumulate excess weight more easily. Instead of foods high in saturated fat, eat more fruits, vegetables, grains, fish, and poultry. As often as possible, eat fresh and homemade foods prepared with a minimum of fats and oils. If you must eat packaged and processed foods, read the labels. Avoid those with a high fat content. Red meat should be used only in small amounts. Avoid recipes that use large amounts of butter, cream, cheese, or other high-fat food in the preparation. Instead, flavor foods with garlic, onions, herbs, lemon juice, or a little olive oil (a monosaturated fat that doesn't increase your cholesterol level). Eat raw seeds and nuts rather than cooked ones (cooking alters the nature of the oils), and use them sparingly because of their high fat content.

Salt. Women with menstrual cramps should carefully avoid excessive salt intake. Too much dietary salt can worsen bloating and fluid retention, thereby contributing to the symptoms of congestive dysmenorrhea. Too much salt intake can also increase high blood pressure and is a risk factor in the development of osteoporosis in menopausal women. Unfortunately, most processed food contains large amounts of salt. Frozen and canned foods are often loaded with salt. In fact, one frozen-food entree can contribute as much as one-half teaspoon of salt to your daily intake. Large amounts of salt are commonly found in the American diet as table salt (sodium chloride), MSG (monosodium glutamate), and a variety of food additives. Fast foods such as hamburgers, hot dogs, french fries, pizza, and tacos are loaded with salt and saturated fats. Common processed foods such as soups, potato chips, cheese, olives, salad dressings, and catsup (to name only a few) are also loaded with salt. And if this were not bad enough, many people use too much salt in their cooking and seasoning.

For women of all ages, I recommend eliminating added salt in your meals. For flavor, use seasonings such as garlic, herbs, spices, and lemon juice. Avoid processed foods that are high in salt, such as canned foods, olives, pickles, potato chips, tortilla chips, catsup, and salad dressings. Learn to read labels and look for the word sodium (salt). If it appears high on the list of ingredients, don't buy the product. Many brands in the health food stores contain foods labeled "no salt added." Some supermarkets also contain "no added salt" foods in their diet or health food section.

Alcohol. Women with menstrual cramps should avoid alcohol entirely or consume it only in small amounts. Alcohol depletes the body's B-complex vitamins and minerals such as magnesium by disrupting carbohydrate metabolism. Because minerals are important in regulating muscle tension, an alcohol-based nutritional deficiency can worsen muscle spasms at the time of menstruation. Depletion of magnesium and B-complex vitamins can also intensify menstrual fatigue and mood swings. Alcohol is toxic to the liver and can affect the liver's ability to metabolize hormones efficiently. Excessive alcohol intake has been associated with lack of ovulation and elevated estrogen levels, which can trigger fibroid growth in susceptible women, thereby worsening menstrual pain. It can also trigger heavy menstrual flow, particularly in women who are transitioning into menopause and have a progesterone deficiency. In women with menstrual cramps, excessive estrogen can worsen the congestive symptoms. Estrogen causes fluid and salt retention in the body. When levels are too high, the body can retain excessive amounts of fluid during the premenstrual and menstrual phases of the month.

When used carefully—not exceeding 4 ounces of wine per day, 10 ounces of beer, or 1 ounce of hard liquor—alcohol can have a delightfully relaxing effect. It makes us more sociable and enhances the taste of food. For optimal health, however, I recommend using alcohol only as an occasional treat, not more than once or twice a week. Women who are particularly susceptible to the negative effects of alcohol shouldn't drink at all.

If you entertain often and enjoy social drinking, I recommend that you try nonalcoholic beverages. A nonalcoholic cocktail such as mineral water with a twist of lime or lemon or a dash of bitters is a good substitute. "Near beer" is a nonalcoholic beer substitute that tastes quite good. Light wine and beer in small amounts have a lower alcohol content than hard liquor, liqueurs, and regular wine.

Sugar. Like alcohol, sugar depletes the body's B-complex vitamins and minerals, which can worsen muscle tension and irritability as well as nervous tension and anxiety.

Unfortunately, sugar addiction is very common in our society among people of all ages. Many people use sweet foods as a way to deal with their frustrations and other upsets. As a result, most Americans eat too much sugar—the average American eats 120 pounds per year. Many convenience foods, such as bottled salad dressing, catsup, and relish, contain high levels of both sugar and salt. Sugar is the main ingredient in soft drinks and in desserts such as candies, cookies, cakes, and ice cream. Highly sugared foods also promote tooth loss through tooth decay and gum disease. Of even greater significance is the fact that excessive sugar intake can worsen diabetes and blood sugar imbalances.

Try to satisfy your sweet tooth instead with healthier foods such as fruit or grain-based desserts, like oatmeal cookies made with fruit or honey. You will find that small amounts of these foods can satisfy your cravings. Instead of disrupting your mood and energy level, they actually have a healthful and balancing effect.

Caffeine. Coffee, black tea, soft drinks, and chocolate—all these foods contain caffeine, a stimulant that many women use to increase their energy level and alertness and decrease fatigue. Caffeine is even used in many over-the-counter menstrual remedies because it does relax blood vessels and promote circulation in the extremities (at the expense of the brain's blood supply). Unfortunately, caffeine has many negative effects on the body. For example, caffeine used in excess increases anxiety, irritability, and mood swings. This can be a real problem for women with anemia who have few emotional and physical reserves. Caffeine also depletes the body's stores of B-complex vitamins and essential minerals, so long-term use can actually increase cramps and menstrual fatigue. Depletion of nutrients like the B-complex vitamins also interferes with carbohydrate metabolism and healthy liver function, which helps to regulate estrogen levels and bleeding. Many menopausal women also complain that caffeine increases the frequency of hot flashes. Coffee, black tea, chocolate, and soft drinks all act to inhibit iron absorption, thus worsening anemia.

How to Substitute Healthy Ingredients in Recipes

Learning how to make substitutions for high-stress ingredients in recipes allows you to use your favorite recipes without compromising your health and well-being. Many recipes start out with ingredients that women with cramps need to avoid, such as dairy products, salt, sugar, chocolate, and wheat. By eliminating the high-stress foods and replacing them with healthier ingredients, you can still make almost any recipe that you choose. For years I have recommended this method to my patients, who have found that they can still have their favorite dishes, but in a much healthier version.

Some women choose to totally eliminate the high-stress ingredients from a recipe. For example, you can make a pasta and tomato sauce but eliminate the Parmesan cheese topping, or a Greek salad without the feta cheese. Some of my patients even make pizza without cheese, layering tomato sauce and lots of vegetables on a pizza crust. In many cases, the high-stress ingredients are not necessary in order to make foods taste good; always remember, they can worsen your symptoms.

If you want to retain a high-stress ingredient, you can substantially reduce the amount of that ingredient while still retaining the flavor and taste. Most of us have palates jaded by too much salt, fat, sugar, and other flavorings. In many dishes, all we taste are the additives; we never really enjoy the delicious flavor of the foods themselves. During the years that I have cooked by substituting low-stress ingredients, I have come to enjoy the subtle taste of the dishes much more. Also, I find that my health and vitality continue to improve with the deletion of high-stress ingredients from my food. Use the following information on how to substitute healthy ingredients in your own recipes. The substitutions are easy and simple to make, and should benefit your health greatly.

How to Substitute for Dairy Products

Decrease the amount of cow's milk cheese you use in food preparation and cooking. If you must use cow's cheese in cooking, decrease the amount by one-half to two-thirds so that it becomes a flavoring or garnish rather than a major source of fat and protein. You can add soft tofu to recipes to replace cheese. I have done this often with lasagna by layering the noodles with tofu and topping with melted soy cheese for a delicious dish. The tofu, which is bland, takes on the taste of the tomato sauce. If you cannot give up cow's milk products, try to use the lower-fat cheeses now available. Goat's or sheep's cheese in small amounts can also replace cow's cheese because the fat they contain is more easily emulsified in the body.

Use soy cheese in food preparation and cooking. Soy cheese is an excellent substitute for cow's milk cheese. It is lower in fat and salt, and the fat it contains isn't saturated. The health food stores offer many brands that come in many different flavors, such as mozzarella, cheddar, American, and jack. The quality of these products keeps improving all the time. You can use soy cheese as a perfect milk cheese substitute in sandwiches, salads, pizzas, lasagnas, and casseroles.

Replace milk in recipes. For cow's milk, substitute potato milk, soy milk, nut milk, or grain milk. Soy milk and nut milk are available at most health food stores. Soy milk is particularly good and comes in many flavors. Many nondairy milks are good sources of calcium and can be used for drinking, eating, or baking. (See the cookbook section in Chapter 5 for an easy way to make an almond-based milk substitute.) One of my personal favorites is a nondairy milk called DariFree that is made from an all vegetable-potato base. It is creamy and sweet and tastes very similar to the best cow's milk, with none of the unhealthy characteristics of dairy products. Even my twelve-year-old daughter likes it. The potato-based milk is high in calcium. It can be found in the dairy section of your local supermarket. It can also be bought dry for easy storage. DariFree can be used exactly as you use cow's milk for beverages, cooking, and baking.

Substitute flax oil for butter. Flax oil is the best substitute for butter that I've found. It is a golden, rich oil that looks and tastes quite a bit like butter. It is delicious used on anything on which you'd normally use butter—toast, rice, popcorn, steamed vegetables, and potatoes. It is extremely high in essential fatty acids—the type of fat that is very healthy for a woman's body. Essential fatty acids help to promote normal hormonal function. Flax oil is quite perishable, however, since it is sensitive to heat and light. You can't cook with it—the food must cook first, and then the flax oil can be added before serving. It also must be refrigerated. I highly recommend using flax oil because of its many health benefits. You can find it in health food stores or can order it through *The LifeCycles Center* if there is no health food store near you.

How to Substitute for Caffeinated Foods and Beverages

Use coffee and tea substitutes. For drinking, the best coffee substitutes are the grain-based beverages like Pero, Postum, and Caffix. Some women may find that discontinuing coffee abruptly is too difficult because of withdrawal symptoms such as headaches. If this is a concern for you, decrease your total coffee intake gradually to one-half to one cup per day. Use coffee substitutes the rest of the time. This will help prevent withdrawal symptoms.

Use decaffeinated coffee or tea as a transition beverage. If you cannot give up coffee immediately, you can start substituting water-process decaffeinated coffee for the real thing. Then try to wean yourself from coffee altogether.

Use herbal teas for energy and vitality. Many women drink coffee for the pick-up they get from it. Those morning cups of coffee allow them to wake up and function through the day. Use ginger instead. It is a great herbal stimulant that won't wreck your health. To make ginger tea, grate a few teaspoons of fresh ginger root into a pot of hot water. Boil and steep. Serve with honey.

Substitute carob for chocolate. Unsweetened carob tastes like chocolate but is far more nutritious. It is a member of the legume family and is high in calcium. You can purchase carob in chunk form as a substitute for chocolate candy or as a powder to be used in baking or drinks. Be careful, however, not to overindulge.

Carob, like chocolate, is high in calories and fat. It should be considered a treat and cooking aid to be used only in small amounts.

How to Substitute for Sugar

Cut the amount of sweetener in your recipes by one-third to one-half. Americans tend to be addicted to sugar. That is a fact based simply on our tendency to consume close to 120 pounds of sugar a year per person. Most of us grew up on highly sugared soft drinks, candy, and rich pastries—no wonder the incidence of diabetes is soaring among our population. I have found that as women decrease their sugar intake, most begin to really enjoy the subtle flavors of the foods they eat.

Substitute concentrated sweeteners. Concentrated sweeteners such as honey and maple syrup have a sweeter taste per quantity used than table sugar. This will allow you to cut down on the actual amount of sugar in a recipe. If you use a concentrated sweetener in place of sugar in an ordinary recipe, reduce the liquid content in the recipe by ¼ cup. If no liquid is used in the recipe, add 3 to 5 tablespoons of flour for each ¾ cup of concentrated sweetener.

Substitute fruit for sugar in pastries. In making muffins and cookies, you may want to try deleting sugar altogether and adding extra fruits and nuts.

How to Substitute for Salt

Substitute potassium-based products for table salt (sodium chloride). Potassium-based products such as Morton's Salt Substitute are much healthier and will not aggravate heart disease or hypertension.

Substitute powdered seaweeds such as kelp or nori to season vegetables, grains, and salads. They are high in essential iodine and trace elements.

Use herbs instead of salt for flavoring. Their flavors are much more subtle and will help even the most jaded palate appreciate the taste of fresh fruits, vegetables, and meats.

Use low-sodium-content liquid flavoring agents. Low-salt soy sauce and Bragg's Amino Acids, a liquid soybean-based flavoring agent, are delicious when used in cooking as salt substitutes. When you add them to soups, casseroles, stir-fries, and other dishes at the end of the cooking process, you will find that you need only a small amount for intense flavoring.

How to Substitute for Wheat Flour

Use whole grain nonwheat flour. Substitute whole grain nonwheat flours, such as rice or barley flour. Whole grain flours are much higher in essential nutrients such as B-complex vitamins and many minerals. They are also higher in fiber content. Rice flour makes excellent cookies, cakes, and other pastries. Barley flour is best used for pie crusts.

How to Substitute for Alcohol

Use low-alcohol or nonalcoholic products for cooking. Substitute low-alcohol or nonalcoholic wine or beer when cooking or preparing sauces and marinades. You will retain much of the flavor that alcohol imparts and you'll decrease the stress factor substantially.

Substitutes for Common High-Stress Ingredients

3/4 cup sugar	1/2 cup honey
	1/4 cup molasses
	1/2 cup maple syrup
	1/2 ounce barley malt
	1 cup apple butter
	2 cups apple juice
1 cup milk	1 cup soy, potato, nut, or grain milk
1 tablespoon butter	1 tablespoon flax oil (must be used raw and unheated)
1/2 teaspoon salt	1 tablespoon miso
	1/2 teaspoon potassium chloride salt substitute
	1/2 teaspoon Mrs. Dash, Spike
	1/2 teaspoon herbs (basil, tarragon, oregano, etc.)
1-1/2 cups cocoa	1 cup powdered carob
1 square chocolate	3/4 tablespoon powdered carob
1 tablespoon coffee	1 tablespoon decaffeinated coffee
	1 tablespoon Pero, Postum, Caffix, or other grain-based coffee substitute
4 ounces wine	4 ounces light wine
8 ounces beer	8 ounces near beer
1 cup white flour	1 cup barley flour (pie crust)
	1 cup rice flour (cookies, cakes, breads)

5

Menus, Meal Plans & Recipes

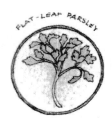

This is one of my favorite chapters because it addresses the pleasure and enjoyment that women can have when preparing and eating health-enhancing foods. My personal interest in meal planning goes back almost 20 years when I first saw the dramatic benefits that a low-stress, high-nutrient diet had on my own menstrual cramps and PMS symptoms. My health problems cleared up beautifully when I made the necessary nutritional changes. I am actually healthier now in my late forties than I was even as a teenager or in my twenties, because I don't have any of the problems that were bothering me then. I give a great deal of the credit for my current excellent health to my continuing emphasis on nutrition. Over the years, I have seen that good nutritional habits have equally beneficial effects on my patients' health problems. Many of my patients have a dramatic reduction in menstrual cramps and congestive symptoms in a very short period of time when they eliminate high-stress foods.

Most of my patients have asked me for specific menus, meal plans, and recipes to help them implement their own self-care program. Unfortunately, very few specific resources are available for women. No cookbooks adequately address a woman's needs for specific nutrients. Most contain recipes that are too high in the nutrients that can worsen cramps, such as animal fats, chocolate, sugar, and salt. More nutrition-conscious cookbooks present low calorie, "light dishes" that eliminate the high-stress ingredients, but still don't give women with menstrual cramps the therapeutic levels of specific nutrients they need. As a result, I've had to develop these resources for women myself.

This chapter contains many menus and recipes that have provided very beneficial therapeutic results for my patients. I have been aware of the busy lives that many women lead and the time demands that so many of us face; thus the recipes are quick, simple, and easy to prepare. I've found that anything too complicated doesn't work for either me or my patients. I use many of these recipes myself since I practice what I preach. Best of all, these recipes are delicious as well as healthy. I hope that you find trying these new dishes to be a delightful adventure as well as beneficial for your health.

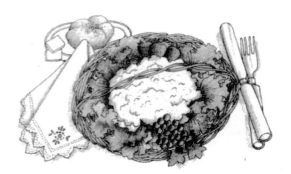

Breakfast Menus

These simple and easy-to-prepare breakfast menus have been developed to reduce and prevent menstrual cramp symptoms. The meal plans and their corresponding recipes do not contain high-stress ingredients. On the positive side, all these dishes contain high levels of the essential nutrients that women with cramps need. I strongly believe that a well-chosen diet can bring therapeutic benefits and have seen this proved with thousands of women over the years.

I have found that breakfast is one of the easiest meals for my patients to restructure along healthier lines. Breakfast is usually eaten at home alone or with family members. It tends to be a smaller and simpler meal. You may want to make healthful dietary changes in your breakfast first and then move on to lunch and dinner.

*Rice cakes
   with raw almond butter
   and fruit preserves
Banana
*Herb tea

*Instant flax cereal
Roasted grain beverage
   (coffee substitute)

*Millet cereal
*Sesame milk

*Rice and oatmeal pancakes
   with flax oil
   and maple syrup
*Herb tea

*Flax shake
Cantaloupe

*Tofu cereal
Prune juice

*Brown rice cereal
Orange juice

*Corn muffins
Raw sesame butter
Roasted grain beverage
   (coffee substitute)

*These recipes are included later in this chapter.

Lunch and Dinner Menus

These menus have been developed to give you a variety of dishes from which to choose when planning your meals. I strongly recommend that you use these menus as helpful guidelines throughout the entire month. Your nutritional status on a day-by-day basis determines how likely you are to have menstrual pain with the onset of each period. These dishes should help to diminish the severity of your cramps because they eliminate high-stress foods.

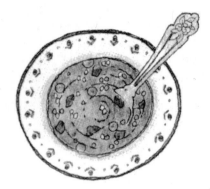

Soup Meals
*Black bean soup
*Corn muffins
*Fresh applesauce

*Carrot soup
*Calcium/magnesium
   vegetable salad
Rye bread and flax oil
Dried figs

*Vegetable soup
Steamed mustard greens
*Baked potato and flax oil
Apple slices

*Tomato-lentil soup
*Broccoli with lemon
*Brown rice
Banana

One-Dish Vegetable Meals
*Vegetarian tacos
   with low-salt salsa

*Tofu and almond stir-fry
Steamed rice

*Pasta with tomato sauce
Green salad

*Hummus
Rye bread
Mixed raw vegetable slices

*Rice and tofu tabouli
Black olives

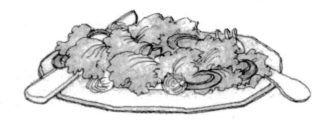

Salad Meals
*Spinach salad
*Corn muffins and flax oil

*Beet salad
Rye muffins
   with fresh fruit preserves

*Calcium/magnesium
   vegetable salad
Rice cakes
Orange slices

*Cole slaw
*Potato salad
Melon

Meat Meals
*Poached salmon
*Brown rice
*Steamed asparagus

*Broiled tuna
*Baked potato with flax oil
*Broccoli with lemon

Broiled trout with dill
Mixed green salad
*Green beans and almonds

Grilled shrimp
Wild rice
*Steamed kale

*These recipes are included later in this chapter.

Breakfast Recipes

Beverages

These drinks utilize specific herbs, fruits, raw seeds, and nuts that have beneficial effects in preventing and treating menstrual cramps. The ingredients contain high levels of essential nutrients that help to relax tension in the muscles of the pelvis and lower extremities. These drinks can also be used throughout the month. Their high mineral and other nutrient content is beneficial for the entire body.

Herb Tea *Serves 2*

1 pint water
1 teaspoon herbs (minced
    ginger root, chamomile
    flowers, peppermint
    leaves, or raspberry leaves)
1 teaspoon honey (if desired)

Bring water to a boil. Place herbs in water and stir. Turn heat to low and simmer for 15 minutes.

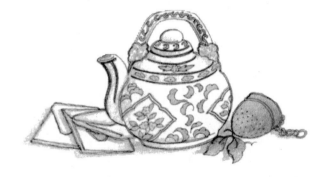

Nondairy Milk Breakfast Shake *Serves 2*

2 cups nondairy milk
2 oz. soft tofu
3 tablespoons flax oil
1 large banana
¾ cup berries (strawberries,
    boysenberries, blueberries,
    or raspberries)

Combine all ingredients in a blender. Blend until smooth and serve. *This delicious, creamy shake is excellent for cramps because it is high in essential fatty acids, calcium, vitamin C, and potassium.*

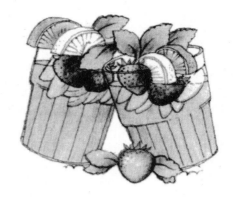

Flax Shake   *Serves 2*

6 tablespoons raw flax seeds

2 bananas

6 oz. water

6 oz. apple juice

Grind flax seeds to a powder using a coffee or seed grinder. Place powdered flax seeds in a blender. Add remaining ingredients and blend. *This recipe is high in essential fatty acids, calcium, magnesium, and potassium because of the whole flax seed.*

Almond Milk   *Serves 1*

½ cup raw almonds

1 tablespoon honey or
    rice syrup

1 cup water

Combine almonds, honey, and ½ cup water in blender. Slowly add remaining water and blend until creamy. If you like a thinner milk, add 1 to 3 ounces more water.

Sesame Milk   *Serves 1*

3 tablespoons raw sesame
    butter or tahini

½ banana

½ cup apple juice

½ cup water

3 ice cubes

Combine all ingredients in blender for a delicious beverage.

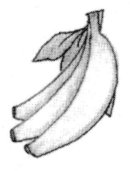

Cereals, Muffins, and Pancakes

Most women have wheat- or dairy-based main courses for break-fast. This includes such commonly used foods as wheat toast, wheat cereal with milk, cottage cheese, and yogurt. As you learned earlier, wheat and dairy products can worsen the symptoms of congestive dysmenorrhea. Diary products are also main triggers for spasmodic dysmenorrhea because they provide the raw mate-rials for the type of prostaglandins that trigger muscle contraction. I have included in this section three types of alternative main dishes you can use to replace wheat and dairy products at break-fast. They are based on whole flax seed and soy- and gluten-free grains. Gluten is the protein found in wheat that can trigger symp-toms of bloating, digestive disturbances, and fatigue.

Instant Flax Cereal

Serves 1

6 tablespoons raw flax seeds

4 to 8 oz. vanilla-flavored nondairy milk

½ banana, sliced

Grind flax seeds to a powder using a coffee or seed grinder. Place powder in a cereal bowl and slowly add nondairy milk, stirring the mixture together. The flax mixture will thicken into a cereal with a texture similar to cream of rice or oatmeal. Top cereal with sliced bananas. Eat the mixture right away because the flax seeds are sensitive to light, air, and temperature. Eat it cold. Do not cook this cereal.

Tofu Cereal

Serves 2

4 ounces soft tofu

2 oz. vanilla-flavored nondairy milk

2 tablespoons flax oil

1 banana

1 apple

15 raw almonds

1 teaspoon honey

Combine all ingredients in a food processor. Blend until creamy. Pour into a bowl and serve. *This is an excellent cereal for cramps because it is high in essential fatty acids, calcium, magnesium, and potassium.*

Millet Cereal #1

Serves 2

1 cup millet

2 cups water

1 teaspoon canola oil

4 oz. vanilla-flavored
nondairy milk

1 tablespoon blackstrap
molasses

1 tablespoon raw
unhulled sesame
seeds

1/2 banana

Wash millet with cold water. Drain. Combine millet, 2 cups water, and canola oil in a cooking pot. Bring ingredients to a boil. Turn heat to low; cover and cook without stirring for 25 to 35 minutes, until millet is soft. Resist temptation to check before 20 minutes, because too much steam will be lost. Fluff up millet and spoon into serving bowls. Add nondairy milk and blackstrap molasses. Top with sesame seeds and banana and serve. *This cereal is extremely high in calcium, magnesium, and potassium. Millet is very high in magnesium, while sesame seeds are high in all three minerals. Blackstrap molasses is a great source of calcium; one tablespoon contains 137 mg of calcium, which is almost 20 percent of the recommended daily allowance.*

Millet Cereal #2

Serves 2

1 cup millet

2 cups water

1 teaspoon canola oil

4 oz. vanilla-flavored
nondairy milk

1 tablespoon honey

3 dried figs, chopped

1 tablespoon sunflower
seeds

Wash millet with cold water. Drain. Combine millet, 2 cups water, and canola oil in a cooking pot. Bring ingredients to a boil. Turn heat to low; cover and cook without stirring about 25 to 35 minutes, until millet is soft. Don't check before 20 minutes, because too much stream will be lost. Fluff up millet and spoon into serving bowls. Add remaining ingredients. Mix and serve. *Figs and raw sunflower seeds are excellent sources of calcium, magnesium, and potassium, which help to relieve cramp symptoms.*

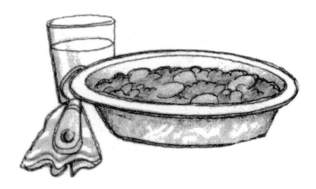

Brown Rice Cereal

Serves 2

1 cup brown rice
2 cups water
1 pinch sea salt
1 oz. raisins
10 raw almonds
1 teaspoon blackstrap
    molasses
2 oz. vanilla-flavored
    nondairy milk or
    apple juice

Wash rice in cold water. Drain. Combine rice, 2 cups water, and salt in a cooking pot. Bring ingredients to a boil. Turn heat to low; cover and cook without stirring about 25 to 35 minutes. Don't lift the lid to check before 20 minutes, because too much steam will be lost. Add remaining ingredients. Mix and serve.

Rice and Oatmeal Pancakes

Serves 4

1¼ cup nondairy milk
1 cup rolled oats
½ cup rice flour
1 tablespoon canola oil
2 eggs, beaten
1 tablespoon honey
1 teaspoon baking powder
1 pinch of salt

Combine nondairy milk, rolled oats, and rice flour and set aside for several minutes. Slowly add canola oil, eggs, honey, baking powder, and salt, mixing as you add each ingredient. Pour mixture onto a lightly oiled hot griddle or frying pan. Cook on medium heat. Turn pancakes when they begin to brown on cooked side and when batter begins to bubble. Serve with maple syrup or fresh fruit preserves.

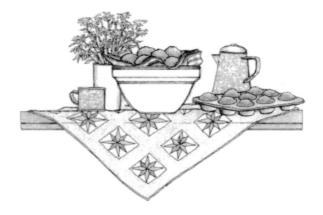

Corn Muffins

Serves 8 to 10

2 tablespoons canola oil

3 tablespoons honey

2 eggs, beaten

2 cups vanilla-flavored nondairy milk

2 cups cornmeal

½ cup rice flour

½ teaspoon salt

1 teaspoon baking powder

½ teaspoon baking soda

Preheat oven to 425°F. Combine oil, honey, eggs, and nondairy milk. Mix well and set aside. In a large bowl, mix cornmeal, rice flour, salt, baking powder, and baking soda. Combine wet and dry ingredients and mix until batter is smooth. Spoon batter into well-oiled muffin tins and bake about 20 minutes. *Muffins are delicious with fresh flax oil (a fine butter replacement), blackberry preserves, or raw almond butter. All these spreads are excellent for cramps.*

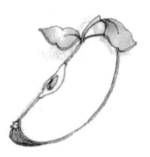

Spreads

These spreads contain highly concentrated levels of ingredients that help to relax muscle tension and relieve congestion. Serve with rice bread, crackers, or corn bread, or even spread on a banana for a delicious treat.

Flax Spread

Serves 2

6 tablespoons raw flax seeds

juice of ½ lemon

½ teaspoon Bragg's Liquid Amino Acids

2 tablespoons water

Grind flax seeds to a powder using a coffee or seed grinder. Place powder in a small bowl. Add the remaining ingredients and mix into a paste. *Use as a spread with rice cakes or crackers.*

Fresh Applesauce

Serves 2

2½ apples

½ cup fresh apple juice

½ teaspoon cinnamon

Peel apples and cut into quarters. Combine all ingredients in a food processor. Blend until smooth.

Lunch and Dinner Recipes

The following dishes do not use red meat, dairy products, poultry, or wheat, all of which can contribute to both congestive and spasmodic dysmenorrhea symptoms. They offer high-nutrient, healthy alternatives that have been developed to help you combat the many symptoms of dysmenorrhea. Mix and match these dishes as you please. You might combine soups and salads or starches and vegetables for a complete meal. The main course dishes are all extremely healthful for women with cramps and can be prepared rapidly. You can use these dishes particularly during the second half of your menstrual cycle, but I recommend using them all month long for optimal health and well-being.

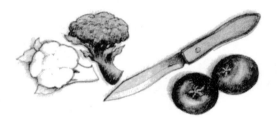

Soups

Black Bean Soup
Serves 4

1 cup black beans
4 cups water
1 onion, chopped
2 cloves garlic, diced
1 carrot, diced
1 potato, diced
2 teaspoons wheat-free soy sauce (tamari)

Wash and drain black beans. Place beans and water in a cooking pot; cover and bring to a boil. Turn heat to low and cook approximately two hours or until beans are tender. Presoaking beans in water overnight will lessen cooking time. (Precooked, canned beans may be used as an alternative.) Add remaining ingredients to soup pot. Bring to a boil; then turn heat to low and cook until beans and vegetables are done.

Carrot Soup

Serves 4

4 cups peeled, sliced carrots
1 1/4 cup diced onions
1/2 cup diced sweet red peppers
4 cups vegetable broth
1 1/2 tablespoon grated gingeroot
1 1/2 cups vanilla non-dairy drink

Combine carrots, onions, red peppers, vegetable broth and ginger in a large pot and cook for thirty minutes or until carrots are tender. Strain out the vegetables and pureé in a food processor. Add vanilla non-dairy milk to blender and pureé together with the soup. Return soup to cooking pot with original broth, stir. Cook on low for five minutes and serve.

Vegetable Soup

Serves 6

4 tomatoes, diced
1 onion, chopped
1 turnip, chopped
1/2 leek, chopped
1 cup peas
2 carrots, chopped
8 mushrooms, sliced
1 bay leaf
1/2 tablespoon thyme
1/2 tablespoon oregano
1/2 teaspoon salt substitute
1 to 1 1/2 quarts water
1/4 bunch parsley, chopped

Place all ingredients except parsley in a pot. Cover with water. Bring to a boil, turn heat to low, cover pot, and simmer for 2 hours. Pour the soup into individual serving dishes. Garnish with chopped parsley.

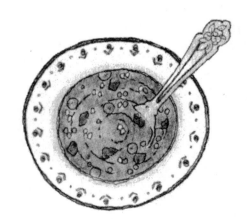

Tomato-Lentil Soup *Serves 4*

1 cup lentils
1/2 onion, chopped
1/2 cup chopped carrots
2 medium tomatoes, diced
1 to 1 1/2 quarts water
1/2 teaspoon wheat-free soy
    sauce (tamari) or salt
    substitute

Wash and drain lentils. Place all ingredients in a pot. Bring to a boil, turn heat to low, cover pot, and simmer for 45 minutes, or until lentils are soft.

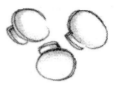

Split Pea and Potato Soup *Serves 4*

1 cup split peas
1/2 onion, chopped
1 medium potato, diced
1/4 to 1/2 teaspoons sea
    salt or salt substitute
1/2 teaspoon oregano
1 quart water

Wash and drain peas. Place all ingredients in a pot; add water. Bring to a boil, turn heat to low, and cover pot. Cook for 45 minutes, or until peas are soft.

Salads

Calcium/Magnesium Vegetable Salad *Serves 4 to 6*

1 head green or red leaf lettuce
1/2 cup chopped steamed
    broccoli
1/2 cup chopped steamed
    green beans
1 small raw carrot, sliced
1 large tomato, sliced
1/4 small red onion, chopped
1/4 cup raw mixed
    bean sprouts

Combine all ingredients in a large salad bowl. Serve with an oil-and-vinegar-based dressing. *Be sure to avoid cheese or cream dressings.*

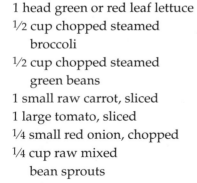

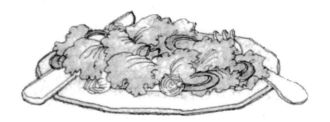

Spinach Salad *Serves 4*

1 bunch spinach, chopped
½ small red onion,
    chopped
⅓ cup diced red pepper
½ cup mung bean sprouts
2 oz. firm tofu, diced
¼ cup raw sunflower seeds

Combine all ingredients in a large salad bowl. Serve with your favorite nondairy dressing.

Beet Salad *Serves 4*

3 medium steamed beets,
    peeled and diced
1 medium red onion,
    chopped
½ bunch parsley, chopped
½ red pepper, diced
¼ cup sunflower seeds

Combine all ingredients in a large salad bowl. Serve with an oil-and-vinegar-based dressing. *Avoid cheese or cream dressing. This salad is great in summer.*

Potato Salad *Serves 6*

8 medium red potatoes
1 cup chopped celery
½ cup finely chopped
    parsley
½ cup chopped green
    pepper
½ cup chopped sweet,
    raw onions

Steam potatoes for approximately 45 minutes. Cool and cube. Combine celery, parsley, pepper, and onions with potatoes; mix thoroughly. Add a small amount of your favorite dressing. *Both vinaigrette and low-calorie mayonnaise are delicious on potato salad.*

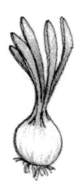

Cole Slaw *Serves 4*

2 cups finely shredded red cabbage

1½ cups finely shredded green cabbage

½ teaspoon celery seeds

½ teaspoon poppy seeds

½ teaspoon dill seeds

Crush or grind seeds and add to shredded cabbage. Serve with favorite dressing (oil-and-vinegar or honey dressing preferred). *The herbs used are high in calcium and magnesium as well as iron.*

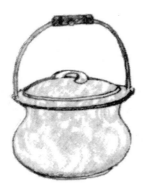

Grains and Starches

Brown Rice *Serves 4*

1 cup brown rice

2 cups cold water

½ teaspoon sea salt

Wash rice with cold water; drain. Combine all ingredients in a cooking pot. Bring to a rapid boil. Turn heat to low, cover, and cook without stirring 25 to 35 minutes or until rice is soft. Resist temptation to check before 20 minutes, because too much steam will be lost.

Kasha *Serves 4*

1 cup kasha (buckwheat groats)

3¼ cups water

pinch of salt

Bring ingredients to a boil. Turn heat to low, cover, and simmer 25 minutes or until soft. The grains should be fluffy like rice. *For breakfast, blend cooked grains in blender with a small amount of water until creamy. Add almond milk, sesame milk, or sunflower milk, and cinnamon, apple butter, ginger, raisins, or berries.*

Baked Potato *Serves 4*

4 russet or Idaho potatoes
1 tablespoon vegetable oil
1 tablespoon flax oil for
   each potato

Preheat oven to 400°F. Wash and dry potatoes, rub them with vegetable oil, and bake 45 to 60 minutes, or until soft when pierced with a fork. Garnish with flax oil. *Other garnishes can include chopped green onions, soy cheese, and low-salt salsa.*

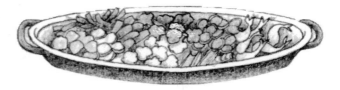

Vegetables

Steamed Asparagus *Serves 4–5*

32 spears asparagus

Separate asparagus tips from lower, tough part of stalks. Discard stalks. Place tips in a steamer with sufficient water to steam for approximately 8 minutes; asparagus should remain bright green. Remove from steamer and serve hot or cold. Use low-calorie mayonnaise or your favorite vinaigrette.

Cauliflower with Flax Oil *Serves 4*

1 medium head cauliflower
4 tablespoons flax oil
1 teaspoon salt substitute

Break the cauliflower into small flowerets. Steam 10 minutes, or until tender. Toss with flax oil and salt substitute and serve.

Broccoli with Lemon *Serves 4*

1 pound broccoli flowerets
juice of 1/2 lemon
4 tablespoons flax oil

Steam broccoli for 12 minutes or until tender. Sprinkle with lemon juice and add flax oil. Mix and serve.

Zucchini and Eggplant

Serves 4

2 medium zucchini, diced
1 cup cubed eggplant
1 small onion, chopped
¾ cup tomato sauce
1 clove garlic, minced
½ teaspoon basil
1 teaspoon oregano

Sauté zucchini, eggplant, and onion at medium heat in a frying pan with a small amount of water. Add remaining ingredients. Cook until tender, stirring constantly.

Steamed Kale

Serves 4

1 bunch kale (stems removed), chopped
juice of 1 lemon
2–3 tablespoons olive oil
pinch of sea salt

Steam kale until tender. Dress with lemon juice, olive oil, and sea salt. *Swiss chard and mustard greens can be prepared and dressed the same way.*

Green Beans and Almonds

Serves 4

1 pound green beans, whole or cut in 2"-pieces
2 oz. raw almonds, chopped
2 tablespoons flax oil
¼ teaspoon salt substitute

Steam green beans until tender. Toss with almond bits, flax oil, and sea salt for a buttery flavor. If you don't care for the taste of flax oil, substitute a vinaigrette.

Whipped Acorn Squash

Serves 4

2 acorn squash
2–3 oz. apple juice
pinch of ground cinnamon

Peel squash and cut into large pieces; steam until tender. Blend in food processor with remaining ingredients until mixture has a smooth consistency.

Steamed Carrots

Serves 4

8 medium carrots, sliced
1 tablespoon maple syrup

Steam carrots until tender. Top with maple syrup and serve.

Main Dishes

Rice and Tofu Tabouli *Serves 6*

2 cups cooked brown rice
1 cup chopped parsley
1/2 cup chopped fresh mint
1/2 medium red onion, diced
1 medium tomato, diced
4 oz. firm tofu, cubed in
    small pieces
juice of 1 lemon
2 tablespoons olive oil
1 teaspoon cumin
1 teaspoon oregano
1/4 teaspoon salt

Combine rice, parsley, mint, red onion, tomato, and tofu. Add lemon juice and olive oil and mix. Add cumin, oregano, and salt to the salad and mix well. *This is the ultimate delicious and healthy tabouli recipe. It is great with the hummus recipe that follows.*

Hummus *Serves 4*

3/4 cup raw unhulled
    sesame seeds
1 cup water or cooking
    liquid from beans
1 3/4 cup cooked
    garbanzo beans
juice of 1 lemon
1 clove garlic
2 tablespoons olive oil
1/4 teaspoon salt

Grind sesame seeds into a powder using a seed or coffee grinder. Place in a dish and set aside. (Raw sesame butter, available from most health food stores, may be substituted). Combine ground sesame seeds, water, garbanzo beans, lemon juice, olive oil, garlic, and salt in a food processor. Blend to the consistency of a smooth dip. Serve as a dip with pita bread, rye bread, and fresh vegetables. *This is great served with rice tabouli (see previous recipe).*

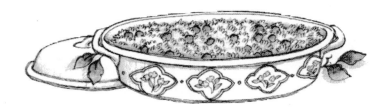

Pesto for Rice and Tofu

Serves 4

2 large cloves garlic, minced

3 cups fresh basil leaves, chopped

1/2 cup almonds, chopped

2 tablespoons grated Parmesan cheese

pinch of sea salt

1/2 cup olive oil

Combine garlic, basil, almonds, cheese, and salt in a food processor until well mixed. Slowly add olive oil until mixture forms a smooth paste. *Pesto may be refrigerated for a few weeks and also freezes well.*

Rice and Tofu

Serves 4

4 cups cooked brown rice

1 cup firm tofu, diced

pesto to taste

Combine rice and tofu in a large bowl. Top with the desired amount of pesto. Mix and serve.

Pasta with Tomato Sauce

Serves 4

1 clove garlic, minced

1/2 small onion, chopped

1/2 green pepper, diced

2 tablespoons canola oil

2 cups chopped tomatoes

1 can (6 oz.) tomato paste

1 teaspoon basil

1 teaspoon oregano

1/2 teaspoon sea salt

1 pound of nonwheat pasta (rice, corn, or buckwheat)

Sauté garlic, onion, and green pepper together in oil over medium heat until tender. Add remaining ingredients, except pasta, and cook on low heat for 15 minutes. In a large pot, cook pasta until it is tender. Drain, place on serving dish, and top with sauce.

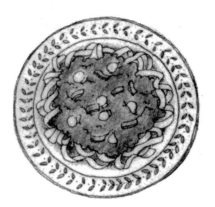

Tofu and Almond Stir-Fry

Serves 4

3/4 cup firm tofu, cubed
1 cup raw almonds, chopped
1/4 yellow onion, chopped
1/2 red pepper, chopped
1/4 cup water
1 teaspoon sesame or
safflower oil
3 cups cooked brown rice
1 teaspoon wheat-free
soy sauce (tamari)

Combine tofu, almonds, onion, and red pepper in a large frying pan with water and oil. Cook over medium heat for 5 minutes. (Add extra water to pan if needed.) Add rice and mix; heat for 5 minutes, or until warm. Transfer to serving dish and toss with wheat-free soy sauce.

Vegetarian Tacos

Serves 4

4 corn tortillas
3/4 pound pinto beans,
cooked and pureéd
1/2 avocado, thinly sliced
1/4 red onion, finely
chopped
1/4 sweet red pepper, diced
1 tomato, diced
6 tablespoons salsa
1/2 head red or romaine
lettuce, chopped

Warm tortillas and beans in separate pans. Place tortillas on individual serving dishes and spread with beans. Garnish with avocado, onion, pepper, and tomato; then cover each taco with lettuce and 1-1/2 tablespoons of salsa.

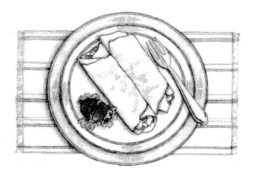

Poached Salmon

Serves 4

4 fillets of salmon, 3 oz. each
1 cup water
juice of 1 lemon

Combine water and lemon juice in skillet and heat. Place salmon in the hot liquid. Cover and poach for 6 to 8 minutes, or until the salmon flakes easily with a fork. Remove the fish and keep it warm until you are ready to serve.

Broiled Tuna *Serves 4*

4 fillets of tuna, 4 oz. each
2 tablespoons lemon juice
1 tablespoon canola oil

Baste fillets with oil; then sprinkle with lemon juice. Place tuna in a broiler pan. Broil for 5 to 6 minutes until fish reaches the level of doneness that you prefer.

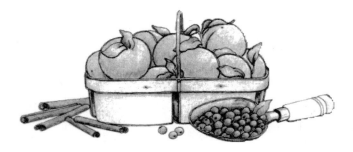

Snacks

Trail Mix *Makes ¾ cup*

4 oz. raw unsalted pumpkin
seeds
4 oz. raw unsalted sunflower
seeds
4 oz. raisins

Combine and store in a container in the refrigerator. *This trail mix recipe is very high in iron and other essential nutrients. I use it to replace stressful and unhealthy sugar-based sweets and chocolate for a snack food. It is a great mix to take on trips and I eat it often for breakfast.*

Rice Cakes with Nut Butter and Jam *Serves 2*

4 unsalted rice cakes
2 tablespoons raw almond
butter
2 tablespoons fruit preserves
(no added sugar)

Spread rice cakes with almond butter and fruit preserves for a quick snack. *Herbal tea makes a good accompaniment.*

Rice Cakes with Tuna Fish

4 unsalted rice cakes
4 oz. tuna fish
2 teaspoons low-calorie
    mayonnaise

Spread rice cakes with tuna fish and mayonnaise. *This is an excellent high-protein/high-carbohydrate snack.*

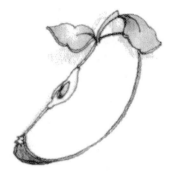

Apple with Almond Butter

1 apple, sliced
1 tablespoon raw almond
    butter

Spread almond butter on apple slices.

Banana with Sesame Butter

1 banana, halved
1 tablespoon raw sesame
    butter

Spread sesame butter on each half of a ripe banana.

Popcorn with Flax Oil

4 oz. popcorn
2 tablespoons flax oil
1/2 teaspoon salt substitute

Popcorn should be hot-air popped into a large bowl. Sprinkle with flax oil and a salt substitute.

6

Vitamins, Minerals & Herbs for Menstrual Cramps

Optimal nutrition plays a crucial role in both the treatment and prevention of menstrual cramps. When adequate nutritional support is lacking, I have found it very difficult to entirely relieve cramp symptoms, even by including powerful drug therapies. Nutrients help relieve cramps in many ways. When used properly, they can promote normal muscle tone and relaxation in the pelvic and low back area. They also help to bring blood circulation and oxygen to the pelvic region. Certain essential nutrients provide the "raw materials" for normal hormone production and balance. In fact, poor or inadequate nutrition may play a major role in causing cramp symptoms. Thus, the use of essential nutrients is an important facet of a good menstrual cramps treatment program. Many research studies done at university centers and hospitals support the importance of nutrition in regulating cramps. I have included a bibliography at the end of this chapter for those wanting more technical information.

The importance of a good diet along with the use of supplements cannot be emphasized too strongly. Supplements are not meant to be used as a rationale to continue poor nutritional habits. I have found that my patients heal most effectively when they combine a nutrient-rich diet with the right mix of supplements. Although nothing can replace a healthful diet, most women have difficulty getting their nutrient intake up to the levels needed for optimal healing through diet alone. The use of supplements can help make up this deficiency so you can heal as rapidly and completely as possible.

This chapter is divided into four sections. The role of vitamins and minerals is discussed in the first section, followed by the beneficial effects of herbs in section two. Section three covers the use of essential fatty acids for menstrual cramps. I complete the chapter with specific recommendations on how to make and use your own supplements. I have also included a number of helpful food charts that give major food sources for each essential nutrient.

Vitamins and Minerals for Menstrual Cramps

This section describes the numerous vitamins and minerals that can be useful in the treatment and prevention of menstrual cramps. Where possible, I have included optimal doses for the nutrients described. You may find, however, that lower doses work better for you. Start slowly when using supplements and increase your dose gradually until you find the level that works best for you.

Vitamin B Complex. The B complex of vitamins consists of eleven factors that work to perform a number of important biochemical functions in the body. These include stabilization of brain chemistry, glucose metabolism, and the inactivation of estrogen by the liver. In fact, vitamin B factors are essential for healthy liver functioning. Emotional and nutritional stress cause loss of the water-soluble B vitamins from the body. Loss of B vitamins can worsen certain symptoms seen with menstrual cramps, including fatigue, faintness, and dizziness. I generally recommend 50 to 100 mg per day of B-complex vitamins. Common food sources of the B-complex vitamins are whole grains, beans and peas, and liver.

Two B vitamins—B_3 and B_6—are particularly useful for menstrual cramps. Niacin, or vitamin B_3, has been shown in clinical research to be effective in relieving 90 percent of menstrual cramps in symptomatic women. The effectiveness of niacin was enhanced with the addition of vitamin C and rutin, a bio-flavonoid. Supplementation needs to be started seven to ten days prior to menses to be effective, and its benefits often remain for several months after stopping its use. Women with pre-existing liver disease should use niacin very cautiously. An optimal dose range for menstrual cramps is 25 to 200 mg per day.

Vitamin B_6, or pyridoxine, can be used to help regulate symptoms of both congestive and spasmodic dysmenorrhea. Clinical studies have shown a reduction in cramping, fluid retention, weight gain, and fatigue with the use of B_6. An interesting clinical study done in 1978 tested the usefulness of vitamin B_6 in decreasing cramps. Women were given vitamin B_6 daily throughout the menstrual period as well as during the rest of the month. Duration and intensity of their cramps decreased progressively over a four- to six-month period. Vitamin B_6 is also an important factor in the conversion of linoleic acid to gamma linolenic acid (GLA) in the production of the beneficial series-one prostaglandins. Prostaglandins have a relaxant effect on uterine muscles, so they can help to reduce cramps. Vitamin B_6 levels are decreased in women using the birth control pill, a common treatment for both spasmodic dysmenorrhea and endometriosis, and should be supplemented. B_6 can be safely used in doses up to 300 mg. Doses above this level can be neurotoxic and should be avoided.

Vitamin C. Vitamin C helps increase capillary permeability. This is important for menstrual cramps since it permits better flow of nutrients into the tight and contracted uterine muscle and facilitates the flow of waste products out of the uterus. Waste products that worsen cramping and pain, such as lactic acid and carbon dioxide, are more efficiently released from the pelvic region. Vitamin C is also an important antistress vitamin and can help decrease the fatigue and lethargy symptoms that accompany cramps. I recommend that women with cramps use from 500 to 3000 mg of vitamin C per day, especially when symptoms occur.

Vitamin E. Vitamin E has been tested in clinical studies as a treatment for spasmodic dysmenorrhea. It has been used in doses of 150 I.U. ten days premenstrual and during the first four days of the menstrual period. It helped to relieve symptoms of menstrual discomfort within two menstrual cycles in approximately 70 percent of the women tested. Vitamin E has a powerful effect on the hormonal system. It has also been used to reduce breast tenderness, fibrocystic disease of the breast, and PMS symptoms, as well as hot flashes in menopausal women. It is obviously a very important nutrient for women's health. The best natural sources of vitamin E are wheat germ oil, walnut oil, soy bean oil, and other grain and seed oil sources. I generally recommend that women with cramps use from 400 to 800 I.U. per day. Women with hypertension and diabetes should start on a much lower dose of vitamin E (100 I.U./day). Any increase in dosage should be made slowly and monitored carefully in these women. Otherwise, vitamin E tends to be extremely safe and is commonly used by millions of men and women.

Calcium. This important mineral helps to prevent menstrual cramps by maintaining normal muscle tone. When taken before bed at night, it is also effective in helping to combat insomnia due to menstrual discomfort. Muscles that are calcium-deficient tend to be hyperactive and more likely to cramp. Since the uterus is made up of muscle, it is susceptible to calcium deficiency. Besides its role in promoting normal muscle tone and activity, calcium is also a major structural component of the bones. Unfortunately, calcium deficiency is common in our society. The recommended daily allowance (RDA) for calcium in menstruating women is 800 mg per day and rises to as much as 1500 mg per day in postmenopausal women. The typical American diet supplies only about 450 to 550 mg per day. No wonder so many American women are at risk for menstrual cramps and osteoporosis. Good food sources of calcium include green leafy vegetables, beans and peas, seeds and nuts, blackstrap molasses, and seafood.

Magnesium. Magnesium has an important effect on the neuro-muscular system in reducing menstrual cramps. Like calcium, a deficiency of magnesium increases muscular hyperactivity. Magnesium actually optimizes the amount of usable calcium in your system by increasing calcium absorption. Conversely, calcium can interfere with magnesium absorption. Magnesium deficiency also worsens menstrual fatigue, dizziness, and fainting because of its importance in glucose metabolism. A magnesium deficiency can hinder the normal conversion of food to usable energy. Magnesium is also needed for the conversion of linoleic acid to gamma linolenic acid (GLA). Like vitamin B_6, a deficiency of magnesium retards the conversion of essential fatty acids to the series-one prostaglandins. Like calcium, magnesium is also an important structural component of healthy bone tissue. It is necessary for the prevention of osteoporosis. It is usually recommended that the diet include half as much magnesium as calcium, or approximately 400 mg per day. Most women get only one-third to one-half of that amount in their daily diet. This puts them at high risk of menstrual cramping and pain.

Iron. Women who have iron deficiency anemia may be at higher risk of menstrual cramps because of the diminished oxygen-carrying capability of the red blood cells. One interesting clinical study showed that when the iron deficiency anemia was resolved, the menstrual cramping disappeared. Young women in their teens and twenties are not only very prone to iron deficiency, but they are also at the peak age for spasmodic dysmenorrhea. Teenagers are prone to heavier menstrual flows during the first few years after they begin menstruation. Also, teenagers and young women in their twenties often eat an iron-poor diet, full of fat and sugar. The RDA for iron is 15 mg. Good food sources of iron include blackstrap molasses, seafood, eggs, liver, vegetables, seeds, nuts, beans, and peas.

Herbs for Menstrual Cramps

A wide variety of herbs will alleviate menstrual cramp symptoms. I have used various cramp-relieving herbs in my practice and many of my patients have found them to be gentle, effective remedies. I use them as a form of extended nutrition, a way of balancing and expanding the diet and optimizing nutritional intake. Some herbs provide an additional source of essential nutrients such as calcium, magnesium, and potassium that help to relieve cramps. Other herbs actually have mild relaxant, diuretic, and anti-inflammatory properties aside from their nutritional content; these help to relieve painful symptoms with a minimum of side effects. In Oriental medicine, cramps are considered a *yang* condition worsened by an excess of foods such as meat and salt. These foods are thought to have a contracting effect on the body. In the traditional Oriental medical practice, cramps are treated by special herbs that have a contrary *yin* effect and cause muscle relaxation and blood vessel dilation. In this section, I describe many specific herbs useful for the reduction of menstrual cramp symptoms.

Sedative Herbs. Herbs such as valerian root, passion flower, hops, and chamomile have a significant calming and restful effect on the central nervous system. They all promote muscle relaxation as well as emotional calm and well-being. With their mild sedative effect, they also promote restful sleep, a state that is difficult to induce when a woman is suffering from menstrual pain. Passion flower has been found to elevate levels of the neurotransmitter serotonin. Serotonin is synthesized from tryptophan, an essential amino acid that has been shown in numerous medical studies to initiate restful sleep. Chamomile, an herb that makes delicate, tasty tea, is a good source of tryptophan. Valerian root has been used extensively in traditional herbal medicine as a sleep inducer and is widely used both in Europe and the United States as a gentle herbal remedy to help combat insomnia. Unfortunately, valerian has an unpleasant taste, making it more palatable when used in capsule form. Both valerian root and chamomile are also effective in relieving indigestion and intestinal gas. Hops and peppermint are other soothing herbs that can be used as teas.

Muscle-Relaxant Herbs. Several Oriental herbs have been used for thousands of years for the treatment of menstrual cramps because they have a direct relaxant effect on the uterine muscle. These herbs are generally available in the United States in health food stores and Oriental herbal shops. Dong Quai, or *angelica sinensis,* is considered an important and effective relaxant herb in Oriental medicine. Angelica root extracts cause an initial increase in uterine tension and contraction, which is then followed by relaxation. Angelica also has significant pain-relieving properties as well, rivaling the effectiveness of aspirin. Peony root is often used in combination with angelica in the treatment of menstrual cramps; it has similar physiological effects on the uterine muscle, but its relaxant effect is more pronounced. Cramp bark is an American herb often used to treat menstrual cramps. It contains high doses of vitamin C and may help to relax the muscle by improving capillary permeability, which aids the flow of essential nutrients to the tense muscle and helps remove the waste products that can worsen cramping, such as lactic acid. Black cohosh, unicorn root, and black haw bark also have a long history in American herbology as effective remedies for menstrual cramps. I have used these herbs often with patients who have subsequently noted significant relief of menstrual discomfort.

Anti-Inflammatory Herbs. White willow has a long and distinguished history as an effective pain reliever in both the Oriental and Western healing traditions. The active painkilling chemical in white willow bark, called salicin, was isolated around 1828 by French and German chemists. Years later, salicylic acid, the precursor of aspirin, was purified. Another natural source of this aspirin precursor was discovered a short time later in the herb meadowsweet. Both meadow-sweet and white willow bark reduce inflammation, pain, and fever. They can be used effectively to help treat menstrual cramps and menstrual headaches since they are able to suppress the action of the series-two prostaglandins. Unfortunately, like aspirin, they can produce the unwanted side effects of gastric indigestion, nausea, and diarrhea, so use these herbs carefully.

Diuretic Herbs. Many herbs act as mild diuretic agents. They can be useful in the treatment of primary congestive dysmenorrhea by reducing bloating and fluid retention. I have used many of them in my practice as mild teas or in tincture form. Some of the most commonly used herbs for congestive symptoms include buchu, celery, dandelion, horsetail, parsley, nettle, sarsaparilla, and uva ursi. All the herbs with diuretic action can deplete your potassium stores on a long-term basis, though they are still much milder than the prescription diuretics. If you use these herbs on a regular basis to treat or prevent primary congestive dysmenorrhea, be sure to eat foods that are high in potassium such as bananas, oranges, raw seeds, and most fruits, as well as nuts and fresh vegetables.

Blood-Circulation Enhancers. Certain herbs such as ginger and ginkgo biloba improve circulation to the pelvis and lower extremities. Ginger causes a widening or dilation of the blood vessels. Better blood circulation helps to draw nutrients to the contracted uterus and low back muscles and also helps to remove waste products like lactic acid and carbon dioxide. Ginger also has an antispasmodic effect on the smooth muscle of the intestinal tract and can help to relieve the digestive symptoms that occur with menstrual cramps, including nausea, vomiting, and bowel changes. Ginger is obviously a useful herb for women with menstrual cramps.

Besides taking ginger in tincture or capsule form, you can also use it as a delicious tea. To make ginger tea, buy a fresh ginger root from your local supermarket. Grate a few teaspoons of the fresh root into a quart pot of water. Boil and steep for 30 minutes.

This is a very soothing herbal tea, delicious with a small amount of honey.

Ginkgo biloba improves blood circulation and oxygenation to the pelvic region and lower extremities. It has a vasodilating effect and also decreases metabolic processes during a period of decreased blood supply. It is a very powerful herbal remedy and can be effectively combined with ginger.

Essential Fatty Acids for Menstrual Cramps

Sufficient essential fatty acids are an extremely important part of the nutritional program for any women with menstrual cramps, whether caused by spasmodic dysmenorrhea or endometriosis. As mentioned earlier in the book, essential fatty acids are the raw materials from which the beneficial hormonelike chemicals called prostaglandins are made. The prostaglandins from essential fatty acids have muscle-relaxant and blood-vessel-relaxant properties that can significantly reduce muscle cramps and tension. There are two essential fatty acids, linoleic acid (Omega 6 family) and linolenic acid (Omega 3 family). They are derived from specific food sources in our diet, primarily raw seeds and nuts, and certain fish including salmon, mackerel, and trout. Linoleic and linolenic acids cannot be made by the body and must be supplied daily in our diets, from either food or supplements. However, once these fatty acids are supplied in the diet, some women may lack the ability to convert them efficiently to the muscle-relaxant prostaglandins. This is particularly true of linoleic acid, which must be converted to a chemical called gamma linolenic acid (GLA) on its way to becoming the series-one prostaglandin.

The conversion of linoleic acid to GLA, followed by the chemical steps leading to the creation of the beneficial prostaglandins, requires the presence of magnesium, vitamin B_6, zinc, vitamin C, and niacin. Women who are deficient in these nutrients can't make the chemical conversions effectively. In addition, women who eat a high-cholesterol diet, eat processed oils such as mayonnaise, use a great deal of alcohol, or are diabetic may find the fatty acid conversion to the series-one prostaglandin difficult to achieve. Other factors that impede prostaglandin production include emotional stress, allergies, and eczema. In women with these risk factors, less than 1 percent of linoleic acid may be converted to GLA. The rest of the fatty acids can be used as an energy source, but they will not be able to play a role in relieving menstrual cramp symptoms.

A number of interesting studies have been done on essential fatty acids as a treatment for PMS. This is particularly relevant for women suffering from menstrual cramps because women with PMS often have the congestive type of dysmenorrhea with bloating, weight gain, and dull aching pain in the pelvic region. Clinical studies have shown that the use of essential fatty acids can reduce most PMS symptoms by as much as 70 percent. Evening primrose oil, borage oil, and black currant oil are the most common supplemental sources of essential fatty acid for the treatment of cramps and PMS. All three oils contain high levels of GLA, allowing women to circumvent the difficult conversion process of linoleic acid to GLA.

The best food sources of essential fatty acids are raw flax seed oil and pumpkin seed oil, which contain high levels of both fatty acids, linoleic and linolenic. Both the seeds and their pressed oils can be used and should be absolutely fresh and unspoiled. Because these oils become rancid very easily when exposed to light and air (oxygen), they need to be packed in special opaque containers and kept in the refrigerator. Fresh flax seed oil is my special favorite. Good quality flax seed oil is available in health food stores. Flax oil is golden, rich, and delicious. It is extremely high in linoleic and linolenic acids, which comprise approximately 80 percent of its total content. Flax oil has a wonderful flavor and can be used as a butter replacement on foods such as mashed potatoes, air popped popcorn, steamed broccoli, cauliflower, carrots, and bread. Flax oil (and all other essential oils) should never be heated or used in cooking, as heat affects the special chemical properties of these oils. Instead, add these oils as a form of flavoring to foods that are already cooked. Pumpkin seed oil has a deep green color and spicy flavor, and is probably more difficult to find than flax seed oil. Eating fresh raw pumpkin seeds provides a good source of this oil. The raw seeds can be purchased from your local health food store and should be kept refrigerated because they are highly perishable. Both flax seed oil and pumpkin seed oil can also be taken in capsule form.

Linolenic acid (Omega 3 family) by itself is found in abundance in fish oils. The best sources are cold-water, high-fat fish such as salmon, tuna, rainbow trout, mackerel, and eel. Linoleic acid (Omega 6 family) by itself can be found in seeds and seed oils. Good sources include safflower oil, sunflower oil, corn oil, sesame seed oil, and wheat germ oil. Many women prefer to use fresh raw sesame seeds, sunflower seeds, and wheat germ to obtain the oils. The average healthy adult requires only four teaspoons per day of the essential oils in their diet, although women with menstrual cramps may need several tablespoons per day of the fresh oil. If you use the whole flax seed, remember that the seeds are 50 percent oil by content, so you need twice as much whole seed intake as oil to obtain the same amount of fatty acids. For optimal results, be sure to use these oils along with vitamin E. The vitamin E also helps to prevent rancidity of the oils.

Nutritional Supplements for Women with Menstrual Cramps

Good dietary habits are crucial for control of your menstrual cramps, but many women must also use nutritional supplements in order to achieve high levels of certain essential nutrients. I have provided two formulas, a vitamin and mineral formula on page 120 and an herbal formula on page 121. These formulas are typical of those that I have frequently used with my patients. You can put these formulas together yourself by combining the individual nutrients. It provides excellent nutritional support for both congestive and spasmodic cramps. You can easily assemble the herbal formula yourself by combining the liquid herbal tinctures in a glass of water.

Remember that all women differ somewhat in their nutritional needs. If you do take the recommended vitamin and mineral or herbal supplements, I usually recommend that you start with one-quarter to one-half of the dose recommended in this book and work your way up slowly to a higher dose level. You may find that you feel best with slightly more or less of certain ingredients to attain the desired results.

I have found that most women can take smaller doses during the time when they are symptom-free. If you use the PMS formulation, two to three capsules per day may be enough to meet your vitamin and mineral needs. During the second half of the cycle when your symptoms occur, double the dose. *Caution:* Do not exceed six to eight capsules per day without the supervision of your physician.

I recommend that patients take all supplements with meals or at least a snack. Very rarely, a woman will have a digestive reaction to supplements, such as nausea or indigestion. If this happens, stop all supplements, then start again, adding one at a time until you find the offending nutrient. Eliminate from your program any nutrient(s) to which you have a reaction. If you have any specific questions, ask a health-care professional who is knowledgeable about nutrition.

Optimal Nutritional Supplementation
For Menstrual Cramps (Daily Doses)*

VITAMINS

Beta carotene	15,000 I.U.
Vitamin B_1 (thiamine)	50 mg
Vitamin B_2	50 mg
Niacinamide	50 mg
Pantothenic acid	50 mg
Vitamin B_6 (pyridoxine HCl)	300 mg
Folic acid	200 mcg
Biotin	30 mcg
Vitamin B_{12}	50 mcg
Choline bitartrate	500 mg
Inositol	500 mg
PABA (para-aminobenzoic acid)	50 mg
Vitamin C	1000 mg
Vitamin D (cholecalciferol)	100 I.U.
Vitamin E	600 I.U.

MINERALS

Calcium (amino acid chelate)	150 mg
Magnesium	300 mg
Iodine	150 mcg
Iron (amino acid chelate)	15 mg
Copper	0.5 mg
Zinc	25 mg
Manganese	10 mg
Potassium	100 mg
Selenium	25 mcg
Chromium	100 mcg

Optimal Herbal Supplements for Menstrual Cramps

(Daily Doses Based upon Herbal Tinctures)

Ginger root	200 mg
White willow bark	200 mg
Chamomile	150 mg
Cramp bark	150 mg
Hops	150 mg
Sarsaparilla	150 mg

Mix dropperfuls of herbal tinctures in a glass of water. You may divide this into a half dose that you use twice a day. Begin use of the herbs one week prior to the onset of your menstrual period.

Food Sources of Vitamin B Complex

Legumes	*Grains*	*Meat, poultry, seafood*
Black beans	Barley	Egg yolks*
Black-eyed peas	Bran	Liver*
Lentils	Corn	
Lima beans	Millet	*Sweeteners*
Pinto beans	Rice bran	Blackstrap molasses
	Wheat	

*Use free-range chickens and animals fed on pesticide-free fodder.

Food Sources of Iron

Grains
Bran cereal (All-Bran)
Bran muffin
Millet, dry
Oak flakes
Pasta, whole wheat
Pumpernickel bread
Wheat germ

Fruits
Apple juice
Avocado
Blackberries
Dates, dried
Figs
Prunes, dried
Prune juice
Raisins

Legumes
Black beans
Black-eyed peas
Garbanzo beans
Kidney beans
Lentils
Lima beans
Pinto beans
Soybeans
Split peas
Tofu

Meat, poultry, seafood
Beef liver
Calf's liver
Chicken liver
Clams
Oysters
Sardines
Scallops
Trout

Vegetables
Beets
Beet greens
Broccoli
Brussels sprouts
Corn
Dandelion greens
Green beans
Kale
Leeks
Spinach
Sweet potatoes
Swiss chard

Nuts and seeds
Almonds
Pecans
Pistachios
Sesame butter
Sesame seeds
Sunflower seeds

Food Sources of Vitamin B6

Grains
Brown rice
Buckwheat flour
Rice bran
Rice polishings
Rye flour
Wheat germ
Whole wheat
　　flour

Vegetables
Asparagus
Beet greens
Broccoli
Brussels sprouts
Cauliflower
Green peas
Leeks
Sweet potatoes

Meat, poultry, seafood
Chicken
Salmon
Shrimp
Tuna

Nuts and seeds
Sunflower seeds

Food Sources of Vitamin C

Fruits
Blackberries
Black currants
Cantaloupes
Elderberries
Grapefruit
Grapefruit juice
Guavas
Kiwi fruit
Mangoes
Oranges
Orange juice
Pineapples
Raspberries
Strawberries
Tangerines

Vegetables
Asparagus
Black-eyed peas
Broccoli
Brussels sprouts
Cabbage
Cauliflower
Collards
Green onions
Green peas
Kale
Kohlrabi
Parsley
Potatoes
Rutabagas
Sweet peppers
Sweet potatoes
Tomatoes
Turnips

Meat, poultry, seafood
Liver—all types
Pheasant
Quail
Salmon

Food Sources of Vitamin E

Vegetables
Asparagus
Cucumber
Green peas
Kale

Nuts and seeds
Almonds
Brazil nuts
Hazelnuts
Peanuts

Meat, poultry, seafood
Haddock
Herring
Mackerel
Lamb
Liver—all types

Oils
Corn
Peanut
Safflower
Sesame
Soybean
Wheat germ

Grains
Brown rice
Millet

Fruits
Mangoes

Food Sources of Essential Fatty Acids

Flax oil
Pumpkin oil
Soybean oil
Walnut oil
Safflower oil
Sunflower oil
Grape oil
Corn oil
Wheat germ oil
Sesame oil

Food Sources of Calcium

Vegetables
Artichokes
Black beans
Black-eyed peas
Beet greens
Broccoli
Brussels sprouts
Cabbage
Collards
Eggplant
Garbanzo beans
Green beans
Green onions
Kale
Kidney beans
Leeks
Lentils
Parsley
Parsnips
Pinto beans
Rutabagas
Soybeans
Spinach
Turnips
Watercress

Meat, poultry, seafood
Abalone
Beef
Bluefish
Carp
Crab
Haddock
Herring
Lamb
Lobster
Oysters
Perch
Salmon
Shrimp
Venison

Fruits
Blackberries
Black currants
Boysenberries
Oranges
Pineapple juice
Prunes
Raisins
Rhubarb
Tangerine juice

Grains
Bran
Brown rice
Bulgar
Millet

Food Sources of Magnesium

Vegetables
Artichokes
Black-eyed peas
Carrot juice
Corn
Green peas
Leeks
Lima beans
Okra
Parsnips
Potatoes
Soybean sprouts
Spinach
Squash
Yams

Meat, poultry, seafood
Beef
Carp
Chicken
Clams
Cod
Crab
Duck
Haddock
Herring
Lamb
Mackerel
Oysters
Salmon
Shrimp
Snapper
Turkey

Nuts and seeds
Almonds
Brazil nuts
Hazelnuts
Peanuts
Pistachios
Pumpkin seeds
Sesame seeds
Walnuts

Grains
Millet
Brown rice
Wild rice

Fruits
Avocados
Bananas
Grapefruit juice
Papayas
Pineapple juice
Prunes
Raisins

Suggested Reading

Castleman, M. *The Healing Herbs*. Emmaus, PA: Rodale Press, 1991.

Erasmus, U. *Fats and Oils*. Burnaby, BC: Alive Books, 1986.

Gittleman, A. L. *Supernutrition for Women*. New York: Bantam Books, 1991.

Hasslering, B., S. Greenwood, M.D., and M. Castleman. *The Medical Self-Care Book of Women's Health*. New York: Doubleday, 1987.

Hogladaroom, G., R. McCorkle, and N. Woods. *The Complete Book of Women's Health*. Englewood Cliffs, NJ: Prentice-Hall, 1982.

Kirschmann, J., and L. Dunne. *Nutrition Almanac*. New York: McGraw-Hill, 1984.

Kutsky, R. *Vitamins and Hormones*. New York: Van Nostrand Reinhold, 1973.

Lambert-Lagace, L. *The Nutrition Challenge for Women*. Palo Alto, CA: Bull Publishing, 1990.

Lark, S., M.D. *Anemia and Heavy Menstrual Flow: A Self Help Program*. Los Altos, CA: Westchester Publishing, 1993.

Lark, S., M.D. *Menopause Self Help Book*. Berkeley, CA: Celestial Arts, 1990.

Lark, S., M.D. *Premenstrual Syndrome Self Help Book*. Berkeley, CA: Celestial Arts, 1984.

Mowrey, D., Ph.D. *The Scientific Validation of Herbal Medicine*. New Canaan, CT: Keats Publishing, 1986.

Murray, M., M.D. *The 21st Century Herbal*. Bellevue, WA: Vita-Line, Inc., 1992.

Padus, E. *The Woman's Encyclopedia of Health and Natural Healing*. Emmaus, PA: Rodale Press, 1981.

Reuben, C., and J. Priestly. *Essential Supplements for Women*. New York: Perigree Books, 1988.

Articles

Abraham, G. E. Primary dysmenorrhea. *Clinical Obstetrics and Gynecology* 1978; 21(1):139–45.

Abraham, G. E. Magnesium deficiency in premenstrual tension. *Magnesium Bulletin* 1982; 1:68–73.

Bauer, U. Six-month double-blind randomized clinical trial of ginkgo biloba extract versus placebo in two parallel groups in patients suffering from peripheral arterial insufficiency. *Arzneim-Forsch* 1984; 34:716–21.

Butler, E. B., and E. McKnight. Vitamin E in the treatment of primary dysmenorrhoea. *Lancet* 1955; 1:844–47.

Fontana-Klaider, H., and B. Hogg. Therapeutic effects of magnesium in dysmenorrhea. *Schweiz Rundsch Med Prax* 1990; 17:79 (16):491–4.

Forman, A., U. Ulmsten, and K. E. Andersson. Aspects of inhibition of myometrial hyperactivity in primary dysmenorrhea. *Acta Obstetrica et Gynecologica Scandinavica* 1983; 113:71–6.

Forster, H. B., H. Niklas, and S. Lutz. Antispasmodic effect of some medicinal plants. *Planta Medica* 1980; 40:309–19.

Gebner, B., A. Voelp, and M. Klasser. Study of the long-term action of a ginkgo biloba extract on vigilance and mental performance as determined by means of quantitative pharmaco-EEG and psychometric measurements. *Arzneim-Forsch* 1985; 35:1459–65.

Glen, I., et al. The role of essential fatty acids in alcohol dependence and tissue damage. *Alcoholism* (NY) 1987; 11(1):37.

Goodnight, S. H. The effects of Omega-3 fatty acids on thrombosis and atherogenesis. *Hematologic Pathology* 1989; 3(1):1.

Gugliano, D., and R. Torella. Prostaglandin E1 inhibits glucose-induced insulin secretion in man. *Prostaglandins and Medicine* 1979; 48:302.

Hanset, A. E., et al. Eczema and essential fatty acids. *American Journal of Disease of Children* 1947; 73:1.

Harada, M., M. Suzuki, and Y. Ozaki. Effect of Japanese angelica root and peony root on uterine contraction in the rabbit in situ. *Journal of Pharmacobio-Dynamics* 1984; 7:304–11.

Hazelhoff, B., T. M. Malingre, and D. K. Meijer. Antispasmodic effect of valeriana compounds: An in-vivo and in vitro study on the guinea pig ileum. *Archives Internationales de Pharmacodynamia* 1982; 257:274–87.

Hernell, Q., et al. Suspected faulty essential fatty acid metabolism in Sjogren-Larrson syndrome. *Pediatric Research* 1982; 16:45.

Hikino, H. Recent research on Oriental medicinal plants. *Economic Medicinal Plant Research* 1985; 1:53–86.

Hindmarch, I., and Z. Subhan. The psychopharmacological effects of ginkgo biloba extract in normal healthy volunteers. *International Journal of Clinical Pharmacology Research* 1984; 4:89–93.

Hollander, D., and A. Tarmawski. Dietary essential fatty acids and the decline in peptic ulcer disease. *Gut* 1986; 22(3):239.

Horrobin, D. F. A biochemical basis for alcoholism and alcohol-induced damage including the fetal alcohol syndrome and cirrhosis: Inter-ference with essential fatty acid and prostaglandin metabolism. *Medical Hypothese* 1980; 6(9):929.

Horrobin, D. F. Essential fatty acids and prostaglandins in metabolism in Sjogren's Syndrome, systemic sclerosis and rheumatoid arthritis. *Scandinavian Journal of Rheumatology Supplement* 1980; 61:242.

Horrobin, D. F. Essential fatty acids and the complications of diabetes mellitus. *Wien Klin Wochenschur* 1989; 101(8):289.

Horrobin, D. F. Essential fatty acids in clinical dermatology. *Journal of the American Academy of Dermatology* 1987; 20(6):1045.

Horrobin, D. F. The regulation of prostaglandins in biosynthesis by the manipulation of essential fatty acid metabolism. *Revue of Pure and Applied Pharmacologic Science* 1980; 4(4):339.

Horrobin, D. F. The role of essential fatty acids and prostaglandins in the premenstrual syndrome. *Journal of Reproductive Medicine* 1983; 28(7):465.

Hudgins, A. P. Vitamins P, C and niacin for dysmenorrhea therapy. *Western Journal of Surgery & Gynecology* 1954; 62:610–11.

Kryzhanovski, G. N., N. L. Luzina, and K. N. Iarygin. Alpha-tocopherol induced activation of the endogenous opioid system. *Biull Eksp Biol Med* 1989; 108(11):566–7.

Kryzhanovski, G. N., L. P. Bakuleva, N. L. Luzina, V. A. Vinogradov, and K. N. Iarygin. Endogenous opioid system in the realization of the analgesic effect of alpha-tocopherol in reference to algomenorrhea. *Biull Eksp Biol Med* 1988; 105(2):148–50.

Luzina, N. L., and L. P. Bakuleva. Use of an antioxidant, alpha-tocopherol acetate, in the complex treatment of algomenorrhea. *Akush Ginekol* (Mosk) 1987; May(5):67–9.

Mieli-Fournial, A. Trace elements in the treatment of dysmenorrhea. *Bulletin de la Federation des Societes de Gynecologie et d'Obstetrique de Langue Francaise* 1968; 20(5):432–3.

Mowrey, D., and D. Clayson. Motion sickness, ginger and psychophysics. *Lancet* 1982; I:655–7.

Penland, J., and P. Johnson. The dietary calcium and maganese effects on menstrual cycle symptoms. *American Journal of Obstetrics and Gynecology* 1993; 168(5):1417-23.

Petkov, V. Plants with hypotensive, antiatheromatous and coronaroldilating action. *American Journal of Clinical Medicine* 1979; 7:197–236.

Puolakka, J., et al. Biochemical and clinical effects of treating the premenstrual syndrome with prostaglandin synthesis precursors. *Journal of Reproductive Medicine* 1985; 39(3):149–53.

Schaffler, V. K., and P. W. Reeh. Double-blind study of the hypoxia-protective effect of a standardized ginkgo biloba preparation after repeated administration in healthy volunteers. *Arzneim-Forsch* 1985; 35:1283–6.

Seifert, B., P. Wagler, S. Dartsch, U. Schmidt, and J. Nieder. Magnesium—a new therapeutic alternative in primary dysmenorrhea. *Zentralbl Gynakol* 1989; 111(11):755–60.

Seltzer, S. Pain relief by dietary manipulation and tryptophan supplements. *Journal of Endodontic* 1985; 11:449–53.

Seltzer, S., D. Dewart, R. Pollack, and E. Jackson. The effects of dietary tryptophan on chronic maxillofacial pain and experimental pain tolerance. *Journal of Psychiatric Research* 1982; 17:181–6.

Shafer, N. Iron in the treatment of dysmenorrhea: A preliminary report. *Current Therapy Research* 1965; 7:365–66.

Somerville, K. W., C. R. Richmond, and G. D. Bell. Delayed release peppermint oil capsules (Colpermin) for the spastic colon syndrome: A pharmacokinetic study. *British Journal of Clinical Pharmacology* 1984; 18:638–40.

Suekawa, M., A. Ishige, K. Yuasa, et al. Pharmacological studies on ginger. I. Pharmacological actions of pungent constituents (6)-gingerol and (6)-shogaol. *Journal of Pharmacobio-Dynamics* 1984; 7:836–48.

Sung, C. P., A. P. Baker, D. A. Holden, et al. Effects of angelica polymorpha on reaginic antibody production. *Journal of Natural Products* 1982; 45:398–406.

Tanaka, S., Y. Ikeshiro, M. Tabata, and M. Konoshima. Anti-nociceptive substances from the roots of angelica acutiloba. *Arzneim-Forsch* 1977; 27:2039–45.

Tanaka, S., Y. Kano, M. Tabata, and M. Konoshima. Effects of "Toki" (Angelica acutiloba Kitagawa) extracts on writhing and capillary permeability in mice (analgesic and anti-inflammatory effects). *Yakugaku Zassh* 1971; 91:1098–1104.

Yamahara, J., T. Yamada, H. Kimura, et al. Biologically active principles of crude drugs. II. Anti-allergic principles in "Shoseiryo-To" anti-inflammatory properties of paeoniflorin and its derivatives. *Journal of Pharmacobio-Dynamics* 1982; 5:921–9.

7

Stress Reduction for Menstrual Cramps

Emotional stress can be a significant trigger for pain, discomfort, and muscle tension. Though we can't always avoid significant stress in our life, we can modify its physical and psychological effects.

The pace of life in Western societies reinforces the tendency toward muscle tension and cramping in sensitive women. To feel rushed and tense is typical in our goal-oriented culture; everything seems to be done in a hurry and on deadlines. We may feel a continual sense of urgency to meet a particular set of goals without giving much attention to how to reach those goals. As a reaction to this sense of urgency, our bodies may tense unconsciously.

Exercises for stress reduction can be a very important part of your menstrual cramp self help program. For many women, the intensity of menstrual cramps varies from month to month. My patients frequently tell me that their cramps are worse when they are more upset. As you begin to anticipate the onset of your menstrual period and cramps, I recommend using stress-reduction techniques on a daily basis. They can really make a difference. If you break up the tasks of the day with a few minutes of stress-reducing exercises, you will feel much more relaxed. With the use of these stress-reduction techniques, you can still accomplish the tasks on time but in a much more relaxed, enjoyable, and health-enhancing manner.

Techniques for Relaxation

To help you deal with the emotional stresses that may become magnified in intensity if you are suffering from menstrual cramps and low back pain, I recommend a variety of relaxation methods. These include focusing, meditation, affirmations, and visualizations. All these methods can help to promote a sense of calm and well-being if practiced on a regular basis. In this chapter, I have included exercises from all these categories for you to try. Choose those you enjoy most and practice them on a regular basis. I have taught these exercises to women patients for many years and love to practice them myself. I usually recommend that my patients learn these techniques on their own through books and tapes, but I sometimes go over the exercises with patients at my office. My patients have been very enthusiastic about the results that they attain through stress-reduction exercises. They often feel much calmer and happier, and also find their physical health is improved. A calm mind seems to have beneficial effects on the body's physiology and chemistry, producing a normalizing effect.

To prepare yourself for the relaxation exercises in this chapter, I suggest that you take the following steps:

First Step. Find a comfortable position. For many women, this means lying on their backs. You may also do the exercises sitting up. Try to keep your spine as straight as possible. Your arms and legs should be uncrossed. It is important that your clothes be loose and comfortable.

Second Step. Focus your attention upon the exercises so that distracting thoughts do not interfere with your concentration. Close your eyes and take a few deep breaths, in and out. This will help to remove your thoughts from the problems and tasks of the day and begin to quiet your mind.

Exercise 1: Focusing

If you have menstrual cramps and low back pain, this focusing exercise allows you to take your attention off the pelvic region and lower part of your body and place your focus elsewhere. By clearing your mind along with doing deep breathing, you may find at the end of this exercise that your discomfort level has diminished in severity.

- Sit upright in a comfortable position.

- Hold several coins, such as 2 quarters, in the palm of your hand.

- Focus all your attention on these coins.

- Inhale and exhale as you do this. Continue to concentrate for 30 seconds. Don't let any other thoughts enter your mind. At the end of this time, notice your breathing. You will probably find that it has slowed down and is calmer. You will probably feel a sense of peacefulness and a decrease in any anxiety that you had before beginning this exercise.

Exercise 2: Discovering Muscle Tension

The next two exercises will help you to get in touch with your own areas of muscle tension and then teach you how to release this tension. This is an important sequence for women with chronic menstrual cramps, low back pain, and abdominal discomfort, because all these symptoms are due in part to chronically tight and tense muscles. Tense muscles tend to have decreased blood circulation and oxygenation and accumulate an excess of waste products such as carbon dioxide and lactic acid. Interestingly enough, some women with cramps and pelvic pain tend to be habitually tense in these areas throughout the month, even during the time when menstrual cramps are absent. Often they have a tendency to tighten the pelvis and lower abdominal muscles as a stress response to a variety of work, relationship, and sexual stresses. Usually, this muscular tensing of the pelvic muscles is an unconscious response that develops over many years and sets up the emotional patterning that triggers cramps.

For example, when a woman has uptight and uncomfortable feelings about sex or a particular sexual partner, she may tighten these muscles when engaging in or even thinking about sex. Tense muscles also affect a woman's moods, making her more "uptight" and irritable. Muscular and emotional tension usually coexist. Movement is one effective way to break up these habitual patterns of muscle holding and contracting. When muscles are loose and limber, a woman tends to feel more relaxed and in a better mood. Anxiety tends to fade away, being replaced by a sense of expansiveness and calm.

- Lie on your back in a comfortable position. Allow your arms to rest comfortably at your sides, palms down, on the surface next to you.

- Now, raise just the right hand and arm and hold it elevated for 15 seconds.

- Notice if your forearm feels tight and tense or if the muscles are soft and pliable.

- Now, let your hand and arm drop down and relax. The arm muscles will relax too.

- As you lie still, notice any other parts of your body that feel tense, muscles that feel tight and sore. You may notice a constant dull aching in certain muscles. Tense muscles block blood flow and cut off the supply of nutrients to the tissues. In response to the poor oxygenation, the muscle produces lactic acid, which further worsens muscular discomfort.

Exercise 3: Progressive Muscle Relaxation

- Lie on your back in a comfortable position. Allow your arms to rest at your sides, palms down, on the surface next to you.

- Inhale and exhale slowly and deeply.

- Clench your hands into fists and hold them tightly for 15 seconds. As you do this, relax the rest of your body. Visualize your fists contracting, becoming tighter and tighter.

- Then let your hands relax. On relaxing, see a golden light flowing into the entire body, making all your muscles soft and pliable.

- Now, tense and relax the following parts of your body in this order: face, shoulders, back, stomach, pelvis, legs, feet, and toes. Hold each part tensed for 15 seconds and then relax your body for 30 seconds before going on to the next part.

- Finish the exercise by shaking your hands and imagining the remaining tension flowing out of your fingertips.

Exercise 4: Healing Meditation

This exercise provides a healing meditation through a series of positive images. The mind and body are inextricably linked. When you visualize a beautiful scene in which your body is being healed, you actually stimulate positive chemical and hormonal changes in your body that help to create this condition. Likewise, if you visualize a negative scene, such as a fight with a spouse or boss, the negative mental picture can actually trigger an output of chemicals from your body that can worsen pain and discomfort. The axiom that we are what we think is literally true. I have seen the power of positive thinking for years in my medical practice. I always tell my patients that it is much harder to heal the body if the mind is full of upsetting, angry, or fearful images. I have found that healing meditations, when practiced on a regular basis, can be a powerful tool for healing.

- Lie on your back in a comfortable position. Inhale and exhale slowly and deeply.

- Visualize a beautiful green meadow full of lovely fragrant flowers. In the middle of this meadow is a golden temple. See the temple emanating peace and healing.

- Visualize yourself entering this temple. You are the only person inside. It is still and peaceful. As you stand inside of this temple, you feel a healing energy fill every pore of your body with a warm golden light. This energy feels like a healing balm that relaxes you totally. All anxiety dissolves and fades from your mind. You feel completely at ease.

- Open your eyes and continue breathing deeply and slowly for a few more cycles.

Exercise 5: Peaceful Meditation

Meditation requires you to sit quietly and engage in a simple and repetitive activity. By emptying your mind, you give yourself a rest. The metabolism of your body slows down. The brain wave slows from the fast beta wave that predominates during our normal working day to a slower alpha or theta wave. This slower pattern is what appears during sleep or in the period of deep relaxation just prior to falling asleep. Meditating gives your mind a break from tension and worry. It is useful to do during menstruation when every little stress is magnified. After meditating you may wonder what all your upset was about. You will see that situations are not as bad as you believed them to be.

- Lie or sit in a comfortable position.

- Close your eyes and breathe deeply. Let your breathing be slow and relaxed.

- Focus all your attention on your breathing. Notice the movement of your chest and abdomen in and out.

- Block out all other thoughts, feelings, and sensations. If you feel your attention wandering, bring it back to your breathing.

- Say the word "peace" as you inhale. Say the word "calm" as you exhale. Draw out the pronunciation of the word so that it lasts for the entire breath. The word "peace" sounds like: *p-e-e-e-a-a-a-c-c-c-e-e-e*. The word "calm" sounds like: *c-a-a-a-l-l-l-m-m-m*. Repeating these two words will help you to concentrate.

♦ Repeat this exercise until you feel very relaxed.

Exercise 6: Affirmations

Affirmations are very important because they align your mind with your body in a positive way. Just as the preceding healing meditation achieved this goal through the use of positive images, affirmations do it through the power of suggestion. Your state of health is determined in part by the interaction between your mind and body via the thousands of messages you send yourself each day with your thoughts. It is not enough to follow an excellent diet and a vigorous exercise routine when you are in the process of healing menstrual cramps. You must tell your body that it is a well, fully functional system. I have seen people stay ill because they sabotage their healing program by sending themselves a barrage of negative messages.

You can aggravate your menstrual cramps and discomfort with negative thoughts because when your body believes it is sick, it behaves accordingly. Thus, it is essential that you cultivate a positive belief system and a positive body image as part of your healing program.

Sit in a comfortable position. Repeat the following affirmations. Repeat those that are particularly important to you 3 times.

- My female system is strong and healthy.

- My hormones are balanced and normal.

- My hormonal levels are perfectly regulated.

- My body chemistry is balanced and normal.

- I go through my monthly menstrual cycle with ease and comfort.
- My body feels wonderful as I start each monthly period.
- I barely know that my body is getting ready to menstruate.
- I feel wonderful each month before I menstruate.
- My uterus is relaxed and receptive; I welcome my monthly period.
- My low back muscles feel supple and pliable with each menstrual cycle.
- I am relaxed and at ease as my period approaches.
- I desire a well-balanced and healthful diet.
- I eat only the foods that are good for my body.
- It is a real pleasure to take good care of my body.
- I love my body; I feel at ease in my body.
- My body is pain-free and relaxed.
- I do the level of exercise that keeps my body healthy and supple.
- I handle stress easily and in a relaxed manner.

Exercise 7: Visualizations

Visualization exercises help you to lay down the mental blueprint for a healthier body. This powerful visual technique can actually stimulate positive chemical and hormonal changes in your body that help create the desired outcome. You are literally imaging your body the way you want it to be. Visualization has been used to great benefit by patients with many types of illnesses. It was pioneered by Carl Simonton, M.D., a cancer radiation therapist, who used this technique with his patients. Instead of seeing their cancers as "big destructive monsters," Dr. Simonton had his patients see their immune systems as big white knights or white sharks attacking the small and insignificant cancer cells and destroying them (instead of the other way around). In a substantial number of cases, he saw his patients' health improve.

Visualization exercises can also help to modify your behavior so that you can create the positive body images that you like. With the practice of visualization, you are more likely to choose your foods carefully and practice regular exercise programs to help your body fit the desired images.

Visualizing the following scene should take a minute or two. Linger on any images that particularly please you.

- Close your eyes. Begin to breathe deeply. Inhale and let the air out slowly. Feel your body begin to relax.

- Imagine that you can look, as if through a magic mirror, deep inside your body.

- Look at your female organs. See your uterus and ovaries. They are an attractive pink color. Your uterus is relaxed and supple. It has good blood circulation. Visualize blood flow and oxygen bringing nourishment to the uterus. See waste products flowing out of the uterus and back into the blood circulation to be removed from the body. See your ovaries. They are extremely healthy and produce just the right levels of hormones. They are shiny and pink and look like two almonds. The fallopian tubes that pick up the eggs and bring them to the uterus are open, elastic, and expandable. They are totally open and healthy.

- Look at your abdominal and low back muscles. They are soft and pliable with a healthy muscle tone. They are relaxed and free of tension during your menstrual period. Your abdomen is flat, yet the area feels relaxed. Your fluid balance is perfect in your pelvic area.

- Look at your entire body and enjoy the sense of peace and calm running through your body. You feel wonderful.

- Now stop visualizing the scene and focus on your deep breathing, inhaling and exhaling slowly.

- You open your eyes and feel very good.

More Stress-Reduction Techniques for Menstrual Cramps

The rest of this chapter contains additional techniques that I have found over the years to be very useful for relaxation of tight and tense muscles. These methods are also useful in inducing deep emotional relaxation. Try them for a delightful experience.

Hydrotherapy

For centuries, people have used warm water as a way to relax muscles and calm moods. You can have your own "spa" at home by adding relaxing ingredients to the bathwater. I have found the following recipes to be extremely useful in relieving muscle pain and tension.

Recipe 1: Alkaline Bath. Run a tub of warm water. Heat will increase your menstrual flow, so keep the water a little cooler if heavy flow is a problem. Add one cup of sea salt and one cup of bicarbonate of soda to the tub. This is a highly alkaline mixture and I recommend using it only once or twice a month. I've found it very helpful in reducing cramps and calming anxiety and irritability. Soak for 20 minutes. You will probably feel very relaxed and sleepy after this bath; use it at night before going to sleep. You will probably wake up feeling refreshed and energized the following day. Heat of any kind helps to release muscle tension. You may also want to try a hot water bottle or a heating pad to relieve cramps.

Recipe 2: Hydrogen Peroxide Bath. This is one of my personal favorites. Hydrogen peroxide is a combination of water and oxygen, so by adding it to your bath, you are using it to "hyper-oxygenate" your bathwater. Hydrogen peroxide is inexpensive and can be purchased from your local drug store. I usually add three pint bottles of the 3-percent solution to a full tub of warm water and soak for up to a half-hour. If you use the stronger food or technical-grade hydrogen peroxide (35-percent strength), you need to add only 6 ounces. With the more concentrated peroxide, be sure to avoid direct contact with your hands or eyes, and keep it stored in a cool place as it is a very powerful oxidizer.

Sound

Music can have a tremendously relaxing effect on our minds and bodies. For women with menstrual cramps and low back pain, I recommend slow, quiet music—classical music is particularly good. This type of music can have a pronounced beneficial effect on your physiological functions. It can slow your pulse and heart rate, lower your blood pressure, and decrease your levels of stress hormones. It can also help to reduce anxiety and induce sleep for women with cramps. Equally beneficial are types of nature sounds, such as ocean waves and rainfall, which can induce a sense of peace and relaxation. I have patients who keep tapes of nature sounds in their cars and at home for use when they feel more stressed. Play relaxing music often as your menstrual cycle approaches and you are aware of increased levels of emotional and physical tension.

Biofeedback Therapy

Biofeedback therapy is an effective way to relieve pain of all kinds caused by muscular tension, as well as poor circulation caused by narrowing of the blood vessel diameter. Constriction of the skeletal muscles and the smooth muscle of the blood vessel wall usually occurs on an unconscious basis, so a person is not even aware it's happening. A variety of factors, including emotional stress and nutritional and chemical imbalances, can trigger this involuntary muscle tension. This constriction can worsen problems such as migraine headaches, high blood pressure, and menstrual cramps.

Biofeedback therapy helps people recognize when they are tensing their muscles. Once this response is understood, menstrual cramp sufferers can learn to relax their muscles to relieve pain. Since muscle relaxation both decreases muscular discomfort and improves blood flow, either factor can be monitored. For relief of cramps, women learn how to implement biofeedback therapy through a series of training sessions. The series usually takes 10 to 15 half-hour office visits with a trained professional. During these sessions, a thermometer is inserted into the vagina like a tampon. The thermometer is connected to a digital readout machine that monitors the woman's internal temperature. The professional teaches her how to consciously change her vaginal temperature. Even a slight rise in the temperature indicates better blood flow and muscle relaxation in the pelvic area, with a concomitant relief of menstrual pain.

After the training sessions, most women are able to raise their temperature at will and thereby control their own cramps. I went through biofeedback training many years ago and found that it had a significant effect on my level of muscle tension. Many hospitals and university centers have biofeedback units, as do stress management clinics, so it is relatively easy to find a treatment facility that offers this type of therapy.

Putting Your Stress-Reduction Program Together

This chapter has introduced many different ways to reset your mind and body to help make menstruation a calm and relaxed time of the month. Try each exercise at least once. Experiment with them until you find the combination that works for you. Doing all seven exercises will take no longer than 20 to 30 minutes, depending on how much time you wish to spend with each one. Ideally, you should do the exercises at least a few minutes each day. Over time, they will help you to gain insight into your negative beliefs and change them into positive new ones. Your ability to cope with stress should improve tremendously.

Suggested Reading

Benson, R., and M. Klipper. *Relaxation Response*. New York: Avon, 1976.

Brennan, B. A. *Hands of Light*. New York: Bantam, 1987.

Davis, M. M., and M. and E. Eshelman. *The Relaxation and Stress Reduction Workbook*. Oakland, CA: New Harbinger Publications, 1982.

Gawain, S. *Creative Visualization*. San Rafael, CA: New World Publishing, 1978.

Gawain, S. *Living in the Light*. Mill Valley, CA: Whatever Publishing, 1986.

Kripalu Center for Holistic Health. *The Self-Health Guide*. Lenox, MA: Kripalu Publications, 1980.

Loehr, J., and J. Migdow. *Take a Deep Breath*. New York: Villard Books, 1986.

Miller, E. *Self-Imagery*. Berkeley, CA: Celestial Arts, 1986.

Ornstein, R., and D. Sobel. *Healthy Pleasures*. Reading, MA: Addison-Wesley, 1989.

8

Breathing Exercises for Menstrual Cramps

Therapeutic breathwork can have a major beneficial impact on menstrual cramps. Through the use of controlled breathing exercises, you can relax and loosen your muscles, decrease sensations of pain, lower your anxiety level, and generate a feeling of internal peace and calm.

When you are breathing slowly and deeply, you take in large amounts of oxygen from the environment. This oxygen is taken into your circulation where it binds to the red blood cells as it travels through the arteries and veins. Oxygen allows the cells to produce and utilize energy as well as help to remove waste products through the production of carbon dioxide. These waste products are cleared through exhalation by the lungs. Thus, the whole body needs optimal levels of oxygen for its normal cycle of building, repair, and elimination.

When you are in physical and emotional distress, oxygen levels are decreased. Breathing tends to become jagged, erratic, and shallow. You may find yourself breathing too fast or with severe pain. You may stop breathing altogether and hold your breath for prolonged periods of time without even realizing it. None of these breathing patterns is healthful. Anxious breathing is often linked to other unhealthy physiological reactions that reflect your body's state of stress. When you have cramps, you tend to tense and tighten your muscles, constrict blood flow, elevate your pulse rate and heartbeat, and stimulate the output of stressful chemicals from your glands as a response to the pelvic discomfort. Waste products such as carbon dioxide and lactic acid also accumulate in your muscles and other tissues.

Therapeutic breathing exercises provide a way to break up this pattern and help the body return to equilibrium. It is important to do the breathing exercises in a slow and regular manner. First, find a comfortable position. Some exercises you should do lying on your back; for other exercises, you'll sit up, uncross your arms and legs, and keep your back straight.

Exercise 1: Deep Abdominal Breathing

Deep, slow abdominal breathing is a very important technique for the relief of menstrual cramps and pain. It brings adequate oxygen, the fuel for metabolic activity, to all tissues of the body. Rapid, shallow breathing decreases oxygen supply and keeps one devitalized. Deep breathing helps to relax the entire body, and strengthens muscles in the chest and abdomen. It also helps calm many other physiological processes, such as rapid pulse rate and heartbeat that often accompany menstrual cramps.

- Lie flat on your back with your knees pulled up. Keep your feet slightly apart. Try to breathe in and out through your nose.

- Inhale deeply. As you breathe in, allow your stomach to relax so that the air flows into your abdomen. Your stomach should balloon out as you breathe in. Visualize your lungs filling up with air so that your chest swells out.

- Imagine that the air you breathe is filling your body with energy.

- Exhale deeply. As you breathe out, let your stomach and chest collapse. Imagine the air being pushed out, first from your abdomen and then from your lungs.

Exercise 2: Peaceful, Slow Breathing

Breathing slowly and peacefully can actually decrease anxiety and help to promote a sense of inner calm and quiet. Such breathing helps our mind to slow down and our emotions to be happier and more harmonious. Life feels good. We make better decisions and relate to those around us in a healthier way when we are calm. Breathing slowly can also calm our physical responses by helping to balance autonomic nervous system function. The autonomic nervous system regulates functions that we're usually not aware of, such as circulation of the blood, muscle tension, pulse rate, breathing, and glandular function.

The autonomic nervous system is divided into two parts that oppose and complement each other, the sympathetic and parasympathetic systems. The sympathetic nervous system is linked to tension and the "fight or flight" response of fear and panic, while the parasympathetic nervous system regulates body responses that are relaxed and calm. When women have menstrual cramps and low back pain, the sympathetic nervous system is in overdrive. The pain sensation causes muscles to tense. Furthermore, the pulse rate tends to accelerate and the blood vessels tend to constrict. Slow, peaceful breathing is a way to calm down these stress responses and bring the body back to a state of balance. By slowing down our breathing, we slow down our other physiologic responses. Our muscles relax and our blood vessels dilate; a state of equilibrium is restored.

- Lie flat on your back with your knees pulled up. Keep your feet slightly apart. Try to breathe in and out through your nose.

- Inhale deeply. As you breathe in, allow your stomach to relax so that the air flows into your abdomen. Let your stomach balloon out as you breathe in. Visualize the lowest parts of your lungs filling up with air.

- Imagine that the air you are breathing in is filled with peace and calm. A sensation of peacefulness and calm is filling every cell of your body. Your whole body feels warm and relaxed as you breathe in this air. Now, exhale deeply. As you breathe out, imagine the air being pushed out from the bottom of your lungs to the top.

- Repeat this sequence until your entire body feels relaxed and your breathing is slow and regular.

Exercise 3: Grounding Breath

When women are in pain and discomfort, they often lose a sense of being grounded, literally rooted to the earth. Some women report a sensation of numbness in their legs and feet. They may say that they feel as if they have no legs at all. The pelvic and low back pain resulting from menstrual cramps causes leg muscles to tighten and decrease blood circulation and oxygenation to lower extremities; this physical response to pain is part of the reason we lose the sense of owning our legs. When we are physically ungrounded, it is very difficult to function mentally; we have a hard time focusing and concentrating. When our bodies are uncomfortable, we may have difficulty working through our projects for the day in a coherent manner. This next breathing exercise will help you to ground and focus both physically and mentally. You should feel much more stable and focused by the end of this exercise.

- Sit upright in a chair. Be sure you are in a comfortable position. Keep your feet slightly apart. Try to breathe in and out through your nose.

- Inhale deeply. As you breathe in, allow your stomach to relax so that the air flows into your abdomen. Let your stomach balloon out as you breathe in. Visualize the lowest parts of your lungs filling up with air. Hold your inhalation.

- See a large, thick cord running from the bottom of your buttocks to the center of the earth. Follow the cord all the way down and see it fasten securely to the earth's center. Run two smaller cords from the bottom of your feet down to the center of the earth also.

- As you exhale, gently push your buttocks into the seat of your chair. Become aware of your buttocks, thighs, calves, ankles, and feet. Feel their strength and solidity.

- Repeat this exercise several times until you feel fully present and grounded.

Exercise 4: Muscle Tension Release Breathing

This exercise will help you to get in touch with and release general muscle tension and tightness. Often when the uterus, abdominal muscles, and low back are tight, we unconsciously tense up muscles throughout the entire body. Often the neck, shoulders, and other vulnerable areas are tense, also. A woman with cramps can have tight and tense muscles in other parts of her body and not even be aware of it. This exercise will help you focus on any tension that you are carrying in your upper body. It will also help you take your focus off your cramps. As you relax and release the muscles in your neck and shoulders, it will help to release muscle tension in your entire body. This is also a good exercise to do while walking or doing sports or desk work, to get in touch with any muscle tension that you may be carrying.

- Sit upright in a chair. Be sure you are in a comfortable position. Keep your feet slightly apart. Try to breathe in and out through your nose.

- Inhale and exhale deeply. As you breathe, let your head move from side to side. Keep your shoulders down and try to touch your ear to your shoulder. As you do this movement, imagine that your neck is made out of putty and that it allows your head to move in a supple, relaxed movement from the left to the right.

- Now inhale and pull your shoulders up towards your ears. Hold your breath and keep your shoulders in a hunched position. Exhale and let your shoulders drop back into a relaxed, comfortable position. Repeat this several times.

- Inhale and exhale deeply as you roll your shoulders forward. Make a large, slow, circular motion with your shoulders. Then, roll your shoulders back slowly. Repeat this several times.

- Inhale and exhale deeply, keeping the rest of your body still and relaxed. Repeat this several times.

Exercise 5: Emotional Cleansing Breath

I have seen, during my years of medical practice, that muscle tension and pain is worse when women are under emotional stress. The more day-to-day stress that you have, involving family, work, and other personal issues, the more this can negatively impact your menstrual cramps. In fact, many of my patients believe that their unhealed family and other personal relations, as well as sexual problems, are significant emotional triggers for their cramps and pain. This exercise uses breathing to help you release any negative feelings, such as chronic anger or upset, that you may be harboring. The more time you spend cleansing old negative emotional patterns, the less impact these feelings can have on your sensitive female reproductive tract with the onset of each menstruation.

- Lie flat on your back with your knees pulled up. Keep your feet slightly apart. Try to breathe in and out through your nose.

- Inhale deeply and see yourself enveloped in a soft white light. Breathe this light into every cell of your body. This is a cleansing light and can help wash away fear, anger, anxiety, and other negative feelings.

- As you exhale deeply, feel the light washing these emotions away.

- Repeat this exercise until you feel emotionally peaceful and clear.

Exercise 6: Color Breathing with Red and Blue

Color breathing has traditionally been used to heal the body and strengthen the body's energy field. Intuitives in our culture can see this energy field as light or colors emanating from the body. When a person is calm, relaxed, and healthy, the energy field appears radiant and full of colors. The colors are bright and harmonious, and each one corresponds to specific parts of the body. When we are feeling pain or tension, which often happens with the chronic symptoms of endometriosis, we lose light and color. Our energy field looks more discordant and jagged, and often the colors change in response to the physical discomfort to duller, more muddied colors. Color breathing is a technique that can help strengthen and heal the energy field as well as the body itself. As you breathe in the healing colors, the parts of your body that are in pain and discomfort often begin to relax and feel healthier again. Tension and cramping is replaced by a sensation of lightness and peace.

- Sit or lie in a comfortable position.

- Take a deep breath and visualize that the earth below you is filled with a deep scarlet red color. This color goes 50 feet below you into the earth. Imagine that you are opening up energy centers on the bottom of your feet. See this color flowing in as you inhale; visualize the deep scarlet red color filling up your feet. Draw this color up your legs and into your pelvic area. See it first filling up your legs, then your lower back, and finally your pelvis. Your uterus is filling with a beautiful deep scarlet red color. As you exhale, see this color flow out of your uterus and lower back and fill the air around you. Exhale the deep scarlet red slowly out of your lungs. Repeat this process 5 times.

- Visualize that the earth is filled with a dark, inky, indigo blue. As you inhale, draw this color into the bottom of your feet. Let it fill your legs, lower back, and pelvic region. See this indigo blue color fill your uterus. As you exhale, see this color flow out of your uterus and lower back and fill the air around you. Exhale the deep indigo blue slowly out of your lungs. Repeat this process 5 times.

Exercise 7: Color Breathing with Golden Light

- Sit or lie in a comfortable position.

- Imagine a cloud of beautiful golden energy surrounding you. As you take a deep breath, inhale the golden energy and visualize it flowing through your body, into your uterus, pelvic area, and lower back. This is a healing energy—it warms and relaxes your uterus, lower abdominal muscles, and lower back.

- Hold the inhalation as long as it is comfortable. Let this golden cloud pick up all your pain and tension.

- Then, exhale this energy out through your lungs and be carried away from you.

- Repeat this process as many times as you need to, until the pain is replaced by a feeling of peace and calm.

9

Physical Exercise for Menstrual Cramps

During my teenage years and through my twenties, I had very few treatment options for my own menstrual cramps. The only treatments available to me were aspirin, heating pads, or bed rest. I often chose the latter and would lie, immobilized with pain, hoping my cramps would stop. During my internship year I began to learn about the importance of lifestyle intervention for the treatment and prevention of menstrual cramps. I began to increase my level of exercise and do more stretching and swimming. I also made significant changes in my dietary habits. Finally, after years of suffering, my menstrual cramps and low back pain started to disappear.

For a number of reasons, exercise promotes pain relief and prevention of menstrual cramps. When women are in pain, they tend to contract their muscles involuntarily. Tight and tense uterine and back muscles have decreased blood flow and oxygenation. Waste products such as excessive carbon dioxide accumulate in this physical environment and can further worsen symptoms. In addition, the pain of menstrual cramps causes breathing to become rapid and shallow. Less oxygen is taken in through respiration, which further decreases the oxygen available to the pelvic region. Metabolism of the muscles becomes less efficient, and fluid retention can become a problem in the pelvic area as well as the ankles and feet. Many women complain of aching pains in their thighs and aching sensations in their legs.

Vigorous aerobic exercise helps to relieve these symptoms of menstrual cramps. Exercise such as tennis, walking, swimming, and dancing requires deep breathing and active movement. Oxygenation and blood flow to the pelvic area improves with better respiration. The vigorous pumping action of the muscles that occurs with these activities helps to reduce the congestive symptoms of menstrual cramps by moving blood and other fluids from the pelvic region.

Exercise also produces significant psychological benefits to cramp sufferers. Improved oxygenation and blood flow benefit the brain as well as the pelvic muscles. The brain demands a healthy share of the body's available nutrients for optimal functioning. When the brain and nervous systems are functioning well, exercise helps to trigger an increased output of endorphins. These are chemicals made by the brain that have a natural opiate effect. Endorphins are thought to produce the "runner's high" that marathoners experience. Many women patients tell me that vigorous exercise is their most effective form of stress management; that exercise produces a sense of peace and relaxation unmatched by anything else they do.

Another way that aerobic exercise might help to reduce anxiety and calm the mood is by helping to balance the autonomic nervous system. The autonomic nervous system regulates the "fight or flight" response that many women experience around the time of their menstrual period. When this system is in overdrive, small life issues can become magnified out of proportion because the body reacts to these small stresses as if they were major life-threatening issues. Regular exercise helps to lessen the intensity of this response.

I also recommend that women with severe menstrual cramps and low back pain consider doing flexibility and stretching exercises as part of their physical activity program. These exercises help to prevent cramps and low back pain by strengthening the back and abdominal muscles. By balancing muscle tension through controlled, slow movement, stretching can also help to improve posture. Stretching exercises demand an awareness of how the parts of the body are aligned spatially with respect to the whole system when the exercises are done properly.

In summary, exercise brings many healthful benefits to women who suffer from menstrual cramps. I recommend that women with cramps follow a regular program of physical activity for cramps throughout the entire month, for both prevention and treatment of this condition. In many ways, exercise is the ideal medicine for women who suffer from menstrual cramps.

General Fitness and Flexibility Exercises for Menstrual Cramps

As part of your self help program, the following exercises will promote mobility, flexibility, and relaxation. You can use them with great benefit during the premenstrual and menstrual time of the month to help loosen the joints in your lower body and decrease muscle stiffness and tension.

You can also do these exercises throughout the month. Practiced on a regular basis, they will improve your vigor and energy level. You can use them to warm up tense and tight muscles before engaging in sports or athletic events.

I do many of these exercises myself and have found them to be very helpful during times of physical and emotional stress and tension. They have helped me tremendously to stay loose and flexible with my own self-care program.

How to Perform the General Fitness and Flexibility Exercises for Menstrual Cramps

- Do all of these exercises during the first week or two of your program. Then put together your own routine based on the exercises that provide the most benefit. You may find that you want to use all of them on a regular basis, or perhaps only a few. Warm-ups should always precede any sports or athletic events.

- The exercises should be performed in a relaxed and unhurried manner. Be sure to set aside adequate time—30 minutes or more—so that you do not feel rushed. Your exercise area should be quiet, peaceful, and uncluttered.

- Wear loose, comfortable clothing. It is better to exercise without socks to give your feet complete freedom of movement and to prevent slipping.

- Evacuate your bowels or bladder before you begin the exercises. Wait at least two hours after eating to exercise.

- Choose a flat area and work on a mat or a blanket. This will make you more comfortable while you do the exercises.

- Pay close attention to the initial instructions when beginning an exercise. Look at the placement of the body as shown in the photographs. This is very important, for you are much more likely to have relief from your symptoms if you practice the exercise properly.

- Try to visualize the exercise in your mind, then follow with proper placement of the body.

- Move slowly through the exercise. This will help promote flexibility of the muscles and prevent injury.

- Always rest for a few minutes after doing the exercises.

- Try to practice these movements on a regular basis. A short session every day is best. If that is not possible, then try to practice them every other day.

Exercise 1: Joint Motion and Flexibility

When women are experiencing an episode of severe uterine cramping with the onset of menstruation, their first instinct is to simply curl up in the fetal position. Often a woman who has menstrual pain will simply stop moving or contract her breathing.

Immobilization is probably the worst thing you can do, because it further cuts off blood flow and oxygenation to the pelvic and low back areas, worsening the pain and tension. Gentle range-of-motion exercises help to loosen tense muscles where they insert and originate near the joints. The following sequence produces a gentle stretching of the muscles around the joints, which will help to reduce tension and stress. These stretches are also thought to stimulate the acupuncture meridians.

- Sit on the floor with your legs stretched out in front. Place your hands at your sides.

- *Toes.* Slowly flex and extend the toes without moving your feet or ankles. Repeat 10 times.

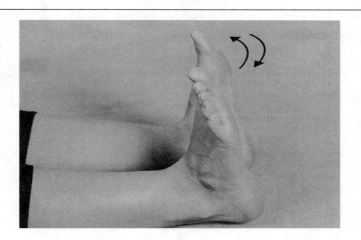

- *Ankles.* Slowly flex and extend the ankle joints. Repeat 10 times.

  Separate your legs slightly, then rotate your ankles in each direction 10 times. Be sure to keep your heels on the floor.

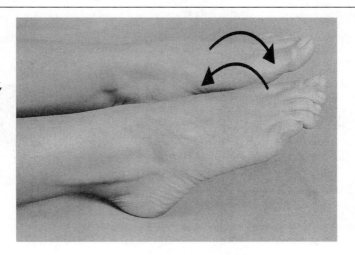

- *Knees.* Still resting in the sitting position, bend the right leg at the knee, bringing the heel near the right buttock.

  Lift the right leg off the ground, straightening the right knee. Repeat 10 times. Then do the same exercise with the left leg.

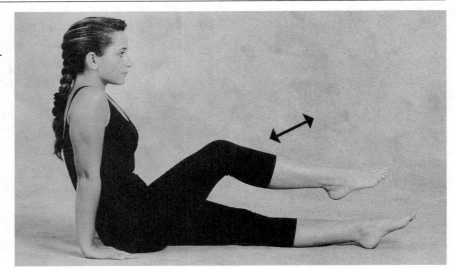

Hold the thigh near the chest with both hands. Rotate your lower leg in a circular motion about the knee 10 times clockwise and then 10 times counter-clockwise. Repeat with the left leg.

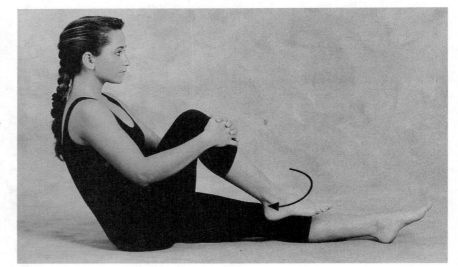

- **_Hips._** Bend the left leg so that you can place your left foot on the right thigh. Hold the left knee with the left hand and hold the left ankle with the right hand. Then gently move the left knee up and down with the left hand. Repeat with the right leg.

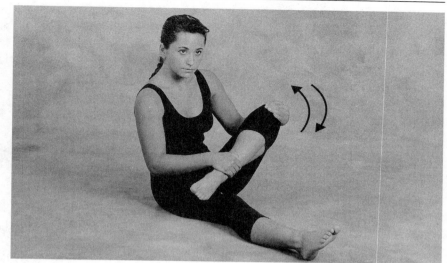

While you are sitting in the same position, rotate the left knee clockwise 10 times and then counter-clockwise 10 times. This improves the flexibility of the hip joints. Repeat on the right side.

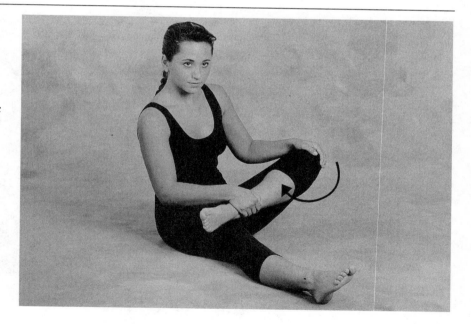

While sitting, bring the soles of the feet together, bringing the heels close to the body. Using the hands, push the knees to the floor and then let them come up again. Repeat 10 times.

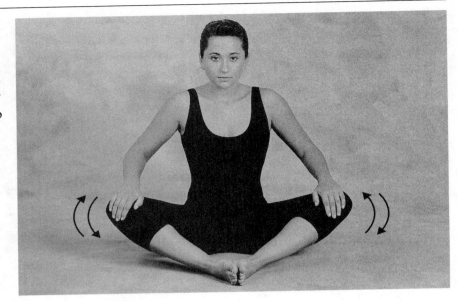

- **Spine.** Remain sitting with your legs together straight in front of you. Reach over and touch your toes without bending your knees. Repeat 20 times.

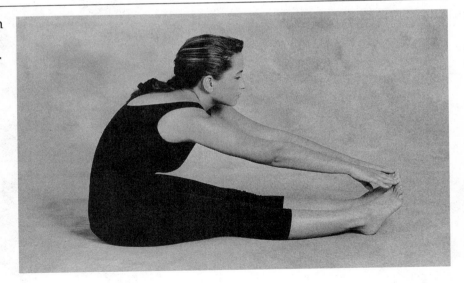

Exercise 2: Muscle Tension Relaxation

This exercise set is excellent for releasing muscle tension and improving circulation in the lower body. It stretches the muscles in the pelvis and lower back. Many women who do this exercise also notice an increase in their energy level. You may have a feeling of vitality upon completing this sequence. The pelvic movements are particularly helpful in bringing optimal blood flow, oxygen, and nutrients to this region, which may help relieve cramps, low back pain, and abdominal tension. Do the steps slowly and never do them so hard as to cause a strain or injury.

- **Legs and Pelvis.** Stand with your legs spread apart about two feet. Point your feet out at a comfortable angle. Bend your knees slowly and lower your buttocks. Eventually, they should be able to go as low as your knees. Move up and down 10 times. Then, rock your pelvis back and forth in a swinging motion.

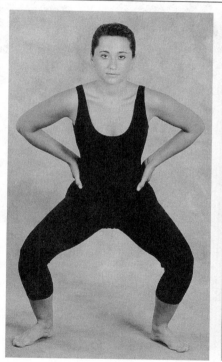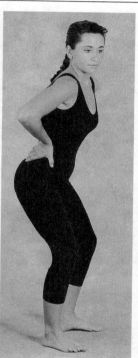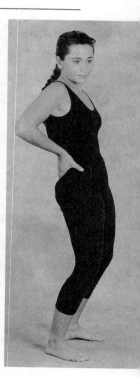

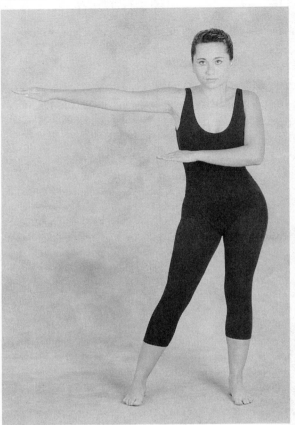 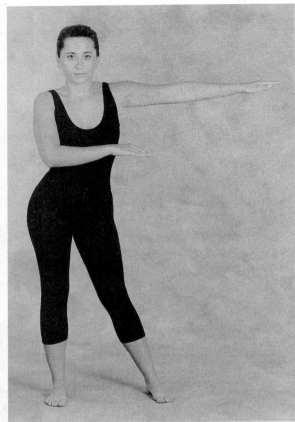

- **Legs and Pelvis.** Move your hips and pelvis from side to side. Let your torso and arms sway in the opposite direction, as if dancing. Then, move your hips around in a full circle. Do this several times in one direction and then the other.

Exercise 3: Lower Back Arch

This exercise helps loosen up the lower back muscles and promotes flexibility of the spine. It can also combat tiredness in women who experience deceased energy during the onset of menstruation.

- Stand with your legs spread apart 1 foot. Point your feet straight ahead.

  Place your hands around your waist with your thumbs pressing into your lower back.

  As you inhale, curve your back into an arch with your head held back. Place your hands around your waist with your thumbs pressing into your lower back.

- As you exhale, let the weight of your body bend you forward so that your head almost touches your knees. Hold for a few seconds.

  Do this exercise slowly and repeat several times.

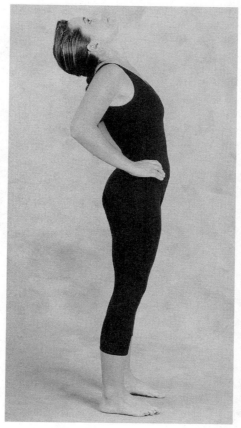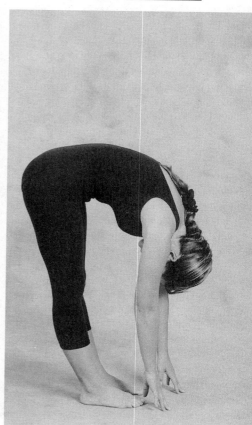

Exercise 4: Abdominal Muscle Release

This exercise helps to release lower and upper abdominal tension. Many women with menstrual cramps often have digestive symptoms such as nausea and bowel changes. This twist helps to reduce the tension in the abdominal muscles that can worsen these symptoms.

- Sit on the floor with your legs crossed. Place your hands on your shoulders with your fingers in front and your thumbs in back. Be sure to keep your spine straight and inhale deeply.

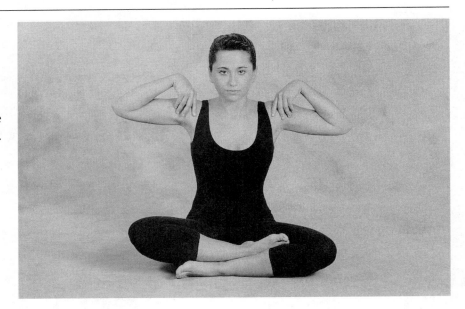

- As you inhale, twist your head, chest, and abdomen to the left. As you exhale, twist your body to the right.

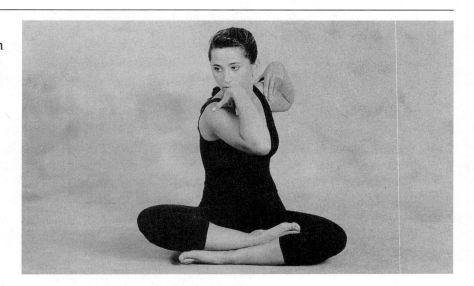

- Do this exercise 4 times. Reverse directions and then repeat the sequence.

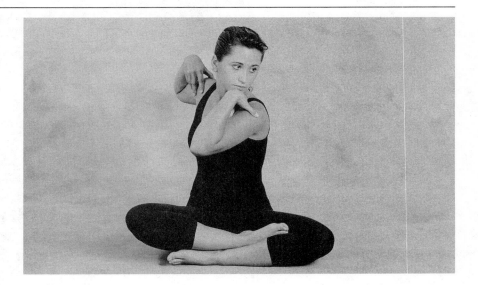

Exercise 5: Low Back Release

This exercise promotes relaxation, specifically in the lower back, hips, and abdominal muscles. By tensing and then releasing the abdominal and hip muscles, along with controlled heavy breathing, the entire mid- and lower body become looser and more supple. You may also notice a decrease in anxiety and emotional tension by the end of this exercise.

- Lie on your back with your legs together. Raise your feet 6 to 8 inches off the ground and then raise your head and shoulders 6 inches, also.

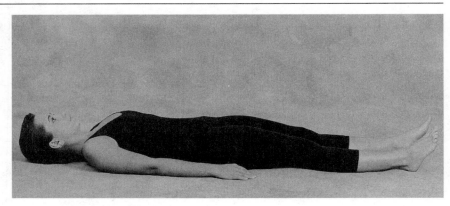

- Point to your toes with your fingertips, keeping your arms straight with your eyes fixed on your toes. Then, breathe through your nose deeply to a count of 20.

- Lower your legs and head and relax.

- Rest for a count of 30.

- Repeat this exercise several times.

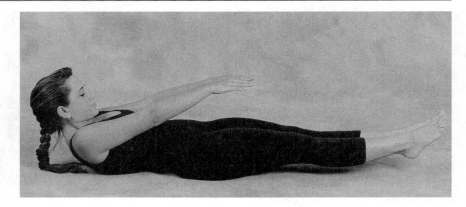

Exercise 6: Low Back Twist

This exercise allows you to twist over to the side, which is actually a natural position for your body to assume when you are feeling pelvic discomfort. This gentle stretch helps to lengthen the muscles in the low back as well as along the entire spine. It also helps to align the lumbar spine. Many women find that this exercise helps relieve pelvic tension and discomfort.

• Lie on your back with your knees bent, feet placed flat on the floor.

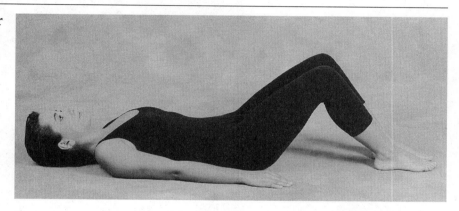

• As you exhale, slowly let your knees and hips fall to the left as you turn your head to the right. Inhale and bring your knees back together to the center.

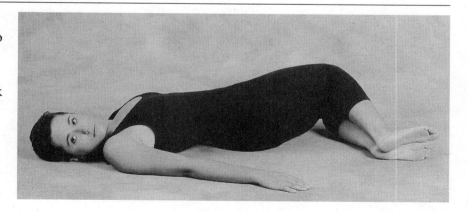

- Then exhale again and reverse direction, letting your knees and hips fall to the right as you turn your head to the left.

- Repeat this exercise slowly several times, alternating sides.

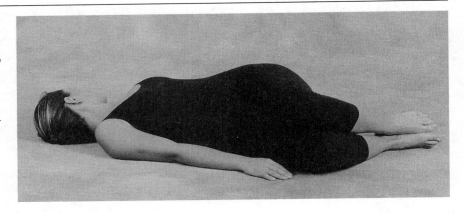

Suggested Reading for Exercise

Caillet, R., M.D., and L. Gross. *The Rejuvenation Strategy*. New York: Pocket Books, 1987.

Hanna, T. *Somatics*. Reading, MA: Addison-Wesley, 1988.

Huang, C. A. *Tai Ji*. Berkeley, CA: Celestial Arts, 1989.

Jerome, J. *Staying Supple*. New York: Bantam Books, 1987.

Kripalu Center for Holistic Health. *The Self-Health Guide*. Lenox, MA: Kripalu Publications, 1980.

McLish, R., and V. Joyce, Ph.D. *Perfect Parts*. New York: Warner Books, 1987.

Pinkney, C. *Callanetics: 10 Years Younger in 10 Hours*. New York: Avon, 1984.

Solveborn, S. A., M.D. *The Book About Stretching*. New York: Japan Publications, 1985.

Tobias, M., and M. Stewart. *Stretch and Relax*. Tucson, AZ: The Body Press, 1985.

10

Yoga for Menstrual Cramps

Yoga stretches can be tremendously beneficial in the treatment and prevention of menstrual cramps, pelvic congestion, and low back pain. The slow, controlled stretching movements that you do in these exercises help to relax tense muscles and improve their suppleness and flexibility. They also help to bring better blood circulation and oxygenation to the tense areas of your lower body, thereby improving the metabolism of the pelvic and back muscles. An additional benefit to yoga is that it helps to quiet your moods. The deep breathing and slow movement that accompany these exercises help to reduce anxiety and irritability and produce a sense of peace.

I have included a series of specific yoga poses that gently stretch every muscle in your body, with specific emphasis on the pelvic and low back region. As well as relieving cramps and discomfort, these exercises energize and balance the female reproductive tract and can help correct underlying hormonal imbalance through improved oxygenation and better circulation to the pelvic area. This can have a beneficial effect on menstrual function. Women who experience fatigue due to menstrual pain and discomfort can enjoy an increase in vigor and stamina when practicing the yoga exercises. I personally do yoga stretches frequently as part of my own exercise routine.

When doing the exercises, it is important that you focus and concentrate on the positions. First your mind visualizes how the exercise is to look, and then your body follows with the correct placement of the pose. The exercises are done through slow, controlled stretching movements. This slowness allows you to have greater control over your body movements. You minimize the possibility of injury and maximize the benefit to the particular part of the body to which your attention is being directed.

Pay close attention to the initial instructions when beginning an exercise. Look at the placement of the body as shown in the photographs. This is very important, for if the pose is practiced properly, you are much more likely to have relief from your symptoms.

I would like to make the following suggestions as you begin these exercises: Try to visualize the pose in your mind, then follow with proper placement of the body. Move slowly through the pose. This will help promote flexibility of the muscles and prevent injury. Follow the breathing instructions provided in the exercise. Most important, do not hold your breath. Allow your breath to flow in and out easily and effortlessly.

If you practice these yoga stretches regularly in a slow, unhurried fashion, you will gradually loosen your muscles, ligaments, and joints. You may be surprised at how supple you can become over time. If you experience any pain or discomfort, you have probably overreached your current ability and should immediately reduce the amount of the stretching until you can proceed without discomfort. Be careful, as muscular injuries can take quite a while to heal. If you do strain a muscle, I have found that immediately applying ice to the injured area for 10 minutes is quite helpful. Continue to use the ice pack two to three times a day for several days. If the pain persists, see your doctor.

Stretch 1: Rock and Roll

This exercise helps to relieve the low back tension that is so common with menstrual cramps. It also massages the neck and spine and flexes the vertebral column. It will invigorate and energize you, reducing fatigue. After doing this exercise, lie flat on your back for a few minutes to enhance the benefits of the exercise.

- Lie on your back. Bend and raise your knees to your chest, clasping them with your hands. Hands should be interlocked below knees.

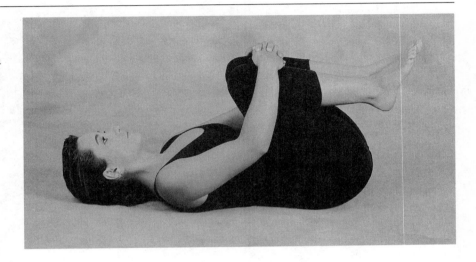

- Raise your head toward your knees and gently rock back and forth on your curved spine. Note the roundness of your back and shoulders. Keep the chin tucked in as you roll back. Avoid rolling back too far on your neck.

- Rock back and forth 5 to 10 times.

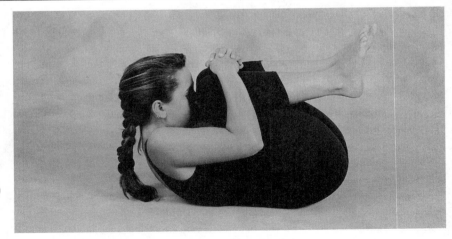

Stretch 2: Pelvic Arch

This is an excellent exercise for stretching the abdominal muscles which are often tightened with menstrual cramps. It is also helpful in reducing pelvic congestion.

- Lie on your back with your knees bent. Spread your feet apart, flat on the floor.

- Place your hands around your ankles, holding them firmly.

- As you inhale, arch your pelvis up and hold for a few seconds. As you exhale, relax and lower your pelvis several times.

- Repeat this exercise several times.

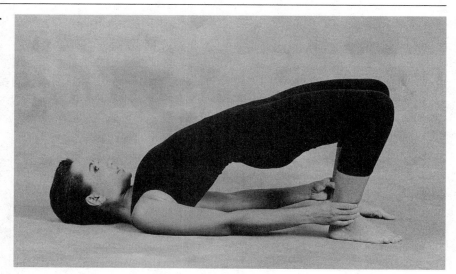

Stretch 3: Cat Cow

This exercise flexes the low back, strengthening this area. By building this area up over time, you can help to prevent menstrual cramps and low back pain.

- Kneel on all fours.

- As you inhale, arch your spine downward while your head goes back.

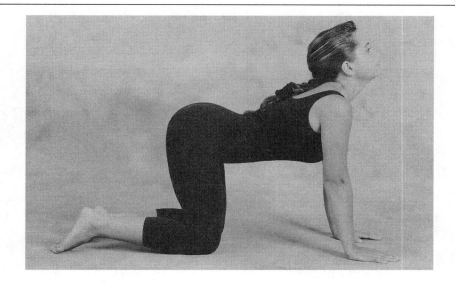

- As you exhale, curve your spine into a rounded arch while your head goes down.

- Do this exercise in a rhythmic, fluid manner.

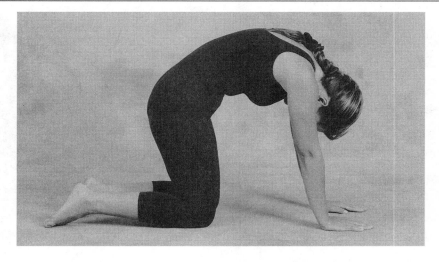

Stretch 4: The Pump

This exercise strengthens the back and abdominal muscles. It also improves blood circulation and oxygenation to the pelvis, which helps to decrease cramps and calms anxiety and nervousness.

- Lie down and press the small of your back into the floor. This permits you to use your abdominal muscles without straining your lower back.

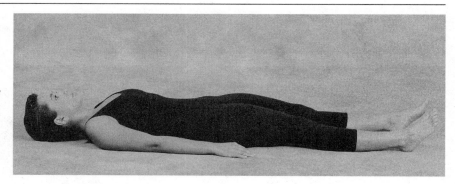

- Raise your right leg slowly while breathing in. Keep your back flat on the floor and let the rest of your body remain relaxed. Move your leg very slowly; imagine your leg being pulled up smoothly by a spring. Do not move your leg in a jerking manner. Hold for a few breaths.

- Lower your leg and breathe out.

- Repeat the same exercise on your left side. Then alternate legs, repeating the exercise 5 to 10 times.

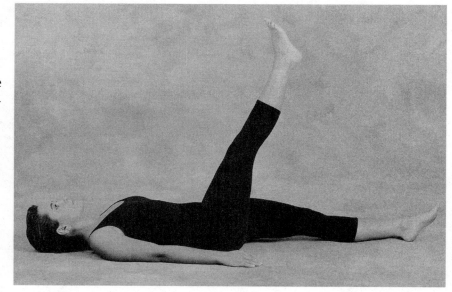

Stretch 5: The Locust

This exercise strengthens the lower back, abdomen, buttocks, and legs and helps to prevent low back pain and menstrual cramps. It also energizes the entire female reproductive tract. Regular practice of this exercise helps to improve posture and elimination. It helps to reduce weight in the thighs and hips and tighten and firm the skin in these areas.

- Lie face down on the floor. Make fists with both your hands and place them under your hips. This prevents compression of the lumbar spine while doing the exercise.

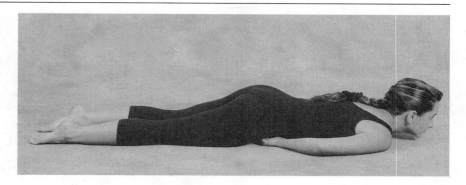

- Straighten your body and raise your right leg with an upward thrust as high as you can, keeping your hips on your fists. Hold for 5 to 20 seconds if possible.

- Lower the leg and slowly return to your original position. Repeat on the left side, then with both legs together. Remember to keep your hips resting on your fists. Repeat 10 times.

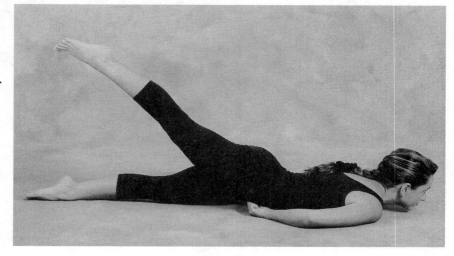

Stretch 6: The Bow

This exercise stretches the entire spine and helps to relieve low back pain and menstrual cramps. It stretches the abdominal muscles and strengthens the back, hips, and thighs. It also stimulates the digestive organs and endocrine glands. Regular practice of this posture can help to relieve depression and fatigue, improving your energy and elevating your mood.

- Lie face down on the floor, arms at your sides.

- Slowly bend your legs at the knees and bring your feet up toward your buttocks.

- Reach back with your arms and carefully take hold of first one foot and then the other. Flex your feet to make grasping them easier.

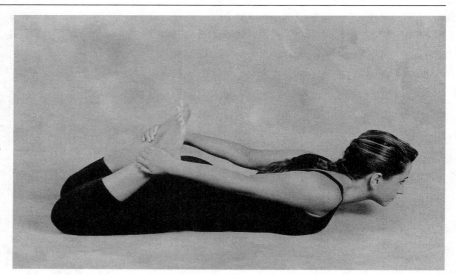

- Inhale and raise your trunk from the floor as far as possible. Lift your head and elevate your knees off the floor.

- Squeeze the buttocks. Imagine your body looking like a gently curved bow. Hold for 10 to 15 seconds.

- Slowly release the posture. Allow your chin to touch the floor and finally release your feet and return them slowly to the floor. Return to your original position. Repeat 5 times.

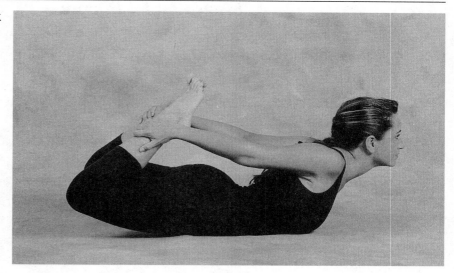

Stretch 7: Child's Pose

This exercise also gently stretches the lower back. It is excellent for calming anxiety and irritability. This is one of the most effective exercises for relieving menstrual cramps.

- Sit on your heels. Bring your forehead to the floor, stretching the spine as far over your head as possible.

- Close your eyes.

- Hold for as long as this is comfortable.

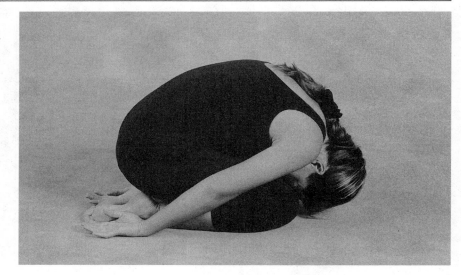

Stretch 8: Wide-Angle Pose

This exercise helps to relieve the congestive symptoms that occur with menstrual cramps. It opens the entire pelvic region and energizes the female reproductive tract. It also relieves bloating and fluid retention in legs and feet.

- Lie on your back with your legs against the wall and extend-ed out like a V or an arc, and your arms extended to the sides.

- Hips should be as close to the wall as possible, buttocks on the floor. Legs should be spread apart as far as they can and still remain comfortable.

- Breathing easily, hold for 1 minute, allowing the inner thighs to relax.

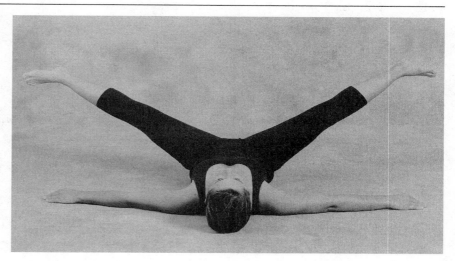

Stretch 9: The Sponge

This exercise relieves menstrual cramps and low back pain. It also relieves anxiety and irritability and reduces eye tension and swelling of the face.

- Lie on your back with a rolled towel placed under your knees. Your arms should be at your sides, palms up.

- Close your eyes and relax your whole body. Inhale slowly, breathing from the diaphragm. As you inhale, visualize the energy in the air around you being drawn in through your entire body. Imagine that your body is porous and open like a sponge, so that this energy can be drawn in to revitalize every cell of your body.

- Exhale slowly and deeply, allowing every ounce of tension to be drained from your body.

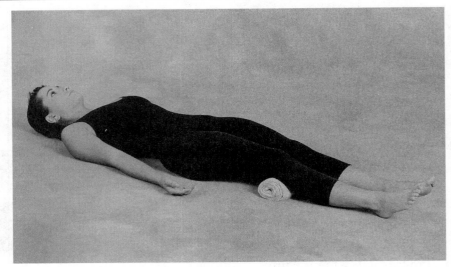

Suggested Reading for Yoga

Bell, L., and E. Seyfer. *Gentle Yoga*. Berkeley, CA: Celestial Arts, 1987.

Couch, J., and N. Weaver. *Runner's World Yoga Book*. New York: Runner's World Books, 1979.

Folan, L. *Lilias, Yoga, and Your Life*. New York: Macmillan, 1981

Mittleman, R. *Yoga 28 Day Exercise Plan*. New York: Workman, 1969.

Iyengar, B. K. S. *Light on Yoga*. New York: Schocken Books, 1966.

Moore, M., and M. Douglas. *Yoga*. Arcane, ME: Arcane Publications, 1967.

Singh, R. *Kundalini Yoga*. New York: White Lion Press, 1988.

Stearn, J. *Yoga, Youth and Reincarnation*. New York: Bantam, 1965.

11

Acupressure for Menstrual Cramps

Acupressure massage is an ancient Oriental healing method that applies finger pressure to specific points on the skin surface to help prevent and treat illness. Acupressure has had a long and distinguished history as an effective healing tool for many centuries and is often used along with herbs to promote the healing of disease.

When specific acupressure points are pressed, they create changes on two levels. On the physical level, acupressure affects muscular tension, blood circulation, and other physiological parameters. On a more subtle level, traditional Oriental healing believes that acupressure also helps to build the body's life energy to promote healing. In fact, acupressure is based on the belief that there exists within the body a life energy called *chi*. It is different from yet similar to electromagnetic energy. Health is thought to be a state in which the chi is equally distributed throughout the body and is present in sufficient amounts. It is thought to energize all the cells and tissues of the body.

The life energy is thought to run through the body in channels called meridians. When working in a healthy manner, these channels distribute the energy evenly throughout the body, sometimes on the surface of the skin and at times deep inside the body in the organs. Disease occurs when the energy flow in a meridian is blocked or stopped. As a result, the internal organs that correspond to the meridians can show symptoms of disease. The meridian flow can be corrected by stimulating the points on the skin surface. These points can be treated easily by hand massage. When the normal flow of energy through the body is resumed, the body is believed to heal itself spontaneously.

Stimulation of the acupressure points through finger pressure can be done by you or by a friend following simple instructions. It is safe, painless, and does not require the use of needles. It can be used without the years of specialized training needed for insertion of needles.

How to Perform Acupressure

Acupressure is done either by yourself or with a friend when you are relaxed. Your room should be warm and quiet. Make sure your hands are clean and nails trimmed (to avoid bruising yourself). If your hands are cold, put them under warm water.

Work on the side of the body that has the most discomfort. If both sides are equally uncomfortable, choose whichever one you want. Working on one side seems to relieve the symptoms on both sides. Energy or information seems to transfer from one side to the other.

Hold each point indicated in the exercise with a steady pressure for one to three minutes. Apply pressure slowly with the tips or balls of the fingers. It is best to place several fingers over the area of the point. If you feel resistance or tension in the area on which you are applying pressure, you may want to push a little harder. However, if your hand starts to feel tense or tired, lighten the pressure a bit. Make sure your hand is comfortable. The acupressure point may feel somewhat tender. This means the energy pathway or meridian is blocked.

During the treatment, the tenderness in the point should slowly go away. You may also have a subjective feeling of energy radiating from this point into the body. Many patients describe this sensation as very pleasant. Don't worry if you don't feel it—not everyone does. The main goal is relief from your symptoms.

Breathe gently while doing each exercise. The point that you are to hold is shown in the photograph accompanying the exercise. All of these points correspond to specific points on the acupressure meridians. You may massage the points once a day or more during the time that you have symptoms.

Acupressure Exercises

Exercise 1: Balances the Entire Reproductive System

This exercise balances the energy of the female reproductive tract and alleviates all menstrual complaints. It also helps relieve low back pain and abdominal discomfort.

Equipment: This exercise uses a knotted hand towel to put pressure on hard-to-reach areas of the back. Place the knotted towel on these points while your two hands are on other points. This increases your ability to unblock the energy pathways of your body.

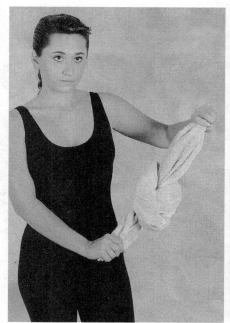
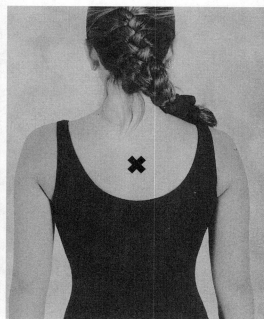

- Lie on the floor with your knees up. As you lie down, place the towel between the shoulder blades on your spine. Hold each step 1 to 3 minutes.

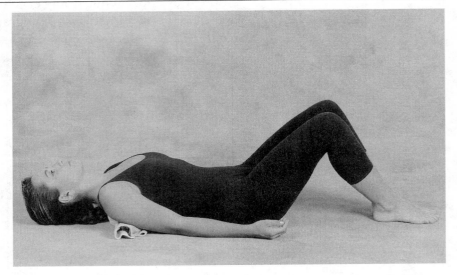

- Cross your arms on your chest. Press your thumbs against the right and left inside upper arms.

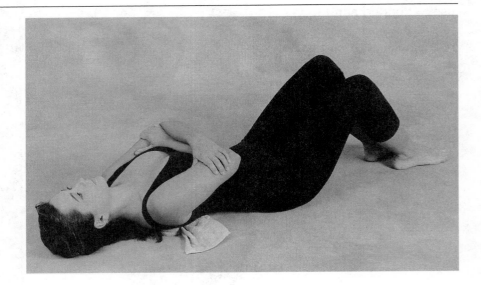

- Left hand holds point at the base of the sternum (breastbone).

  Right hand holds point at the base of the head (at the junction of the spine and the skull).

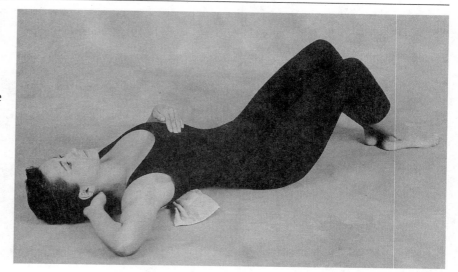

- Interlace your fingers. Place them below your breasts. Fingertips should press directly against the body.

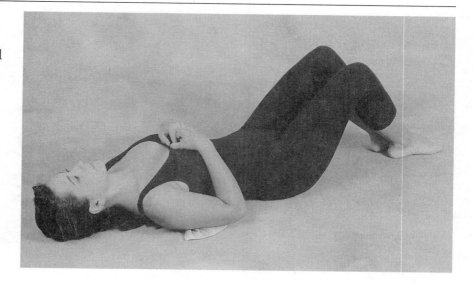

- Move the knotted towel along the spine to the waistline.

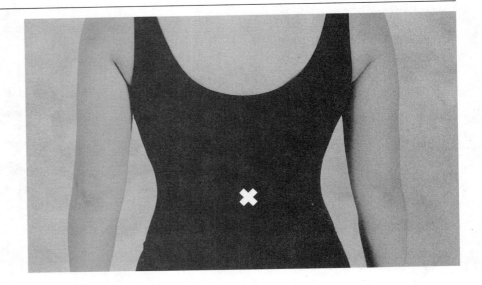

Left hand should be placed at the top of the pubic bone, pressing down.

Right hand holds point on tailbone.

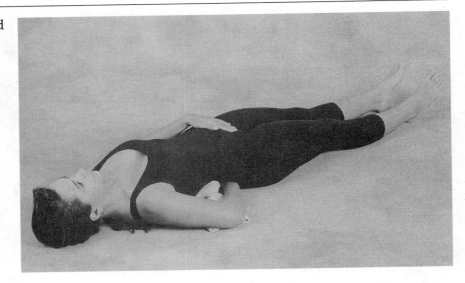

Exercise 2: Relieves Cramps, Bloating, Fluid Retention, Weight Gain

This sequence of points balances the points on the spleen meridian. It helps to relieve menstrual cramps. It also relieves bloating and fluid retention and helps to minimize weight gain in the period leading up to menstruation.

- Sit up and prop your back against a chair, or lie down and put your lower legs on a chair. Hold each step 1 to 3 minutes.

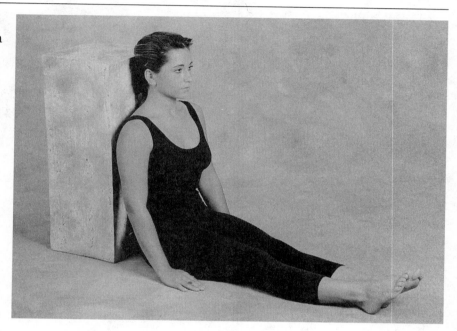

- Left hand is placed in the crease of the groin where you bend your leg, one-third to one-half way between the hip bone and the outside edge of the pubic bone. Right hand holds a spot 2 to 3 inches above the knee.

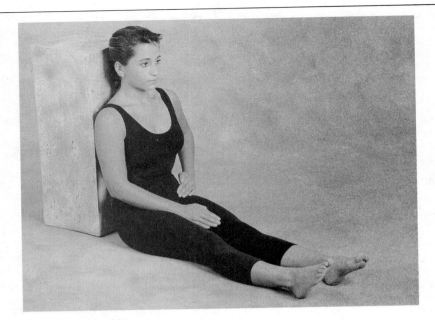

- Left hand remains in the crease of the groin.

  Right hand holds point below inner part of knee. To find the point, follow the curve of the bone just below the knee. Hold the underside of the curve with your fingers.

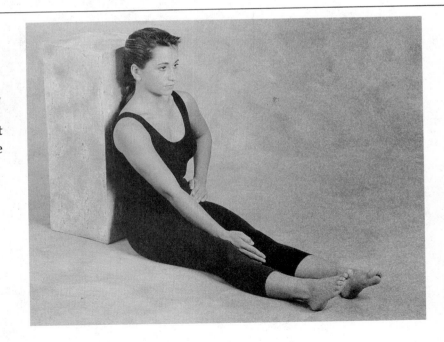

- Left hand remains in the crease of the groin.

  Right hand holds the inside of the shin. To find this point, go four fingerwidths above the ankle bone. The point is just above the top finger.

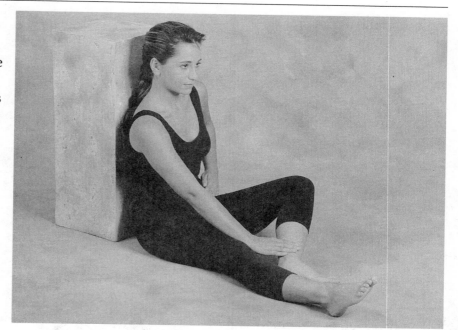

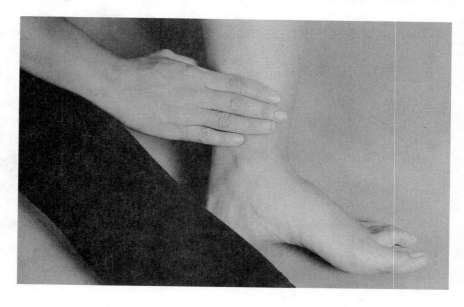

- Left hand remains in the crease of the groin.

  Right hand holds the edge of the instep. To find the point, follow the big toe bone up until you hit a knobby, prominent small bone.

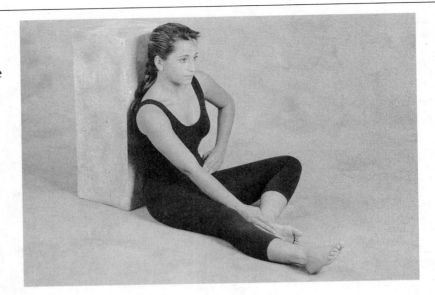

- Left hand remains in the crease of the groin.

  Right hand holds the big toe over the nail, front and back of the toe.

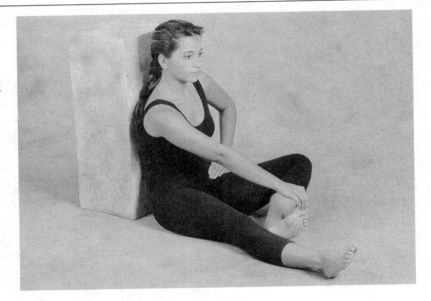

Exercise 3: Relieves Nausea

This exercise relieves the nausea and digestive symptoms that often occur with cramps and low back pain.

- Lie on the floor or sit up. Hold the points 1 to 3 minutes.

- Left index finger is placed in navel and pointed slightly toward the head.

  Right hand holds point at the base of the head.

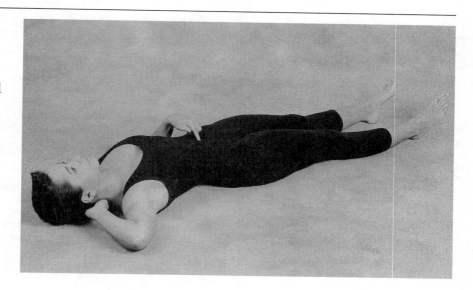

Exercise 4: Relieves Menstrual Fatigue

This sequence of points relieves the fatigue that women experience just prior to the onset of their menstrual period. Tiredness may last through the first few days of menstruation for many women. This exercise can also help to relieve menstrual anxiety and depression. Caution: The second step in this sequence has traditionally been forbidden for use by pregnant women after their first trimester.

- Sit up and prop your back against a chair. Hold each step 1 to 3 minutes.

- Left hand holds point at the base of the ball of the left foot. This point is located between the two pads of the foot.

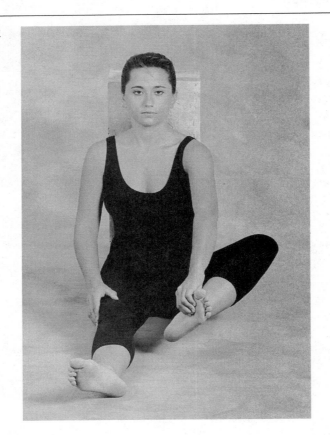

- Right hand holds the point midway between the inside of the right ankle-bone and the Achilles tendon. The Achilles tendon is located at the back of the ankle.

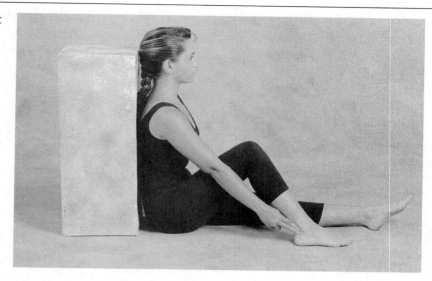

- Left hand holds point below right knee. This point is located four fingerwidths below the kneecap toward the outside of the shinbone. It is sensitive to the touch in many people.

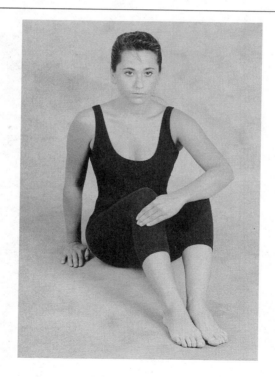

Exercise 5: Relieves Low Back Pain and Cramps

This exercise relieves menstrual cramps and low back pain by balancing points on the bladder meridian. It also balances the energy of the female reproductive tract.

- Sit on the floor and prop your back against a wall or a heavy piece of furniture. Hold each step 1 to 3 minutes.

- Alternative Method: Lie on the floor and put your lower legs over the seat of a chair. Follow the exercise from that position.

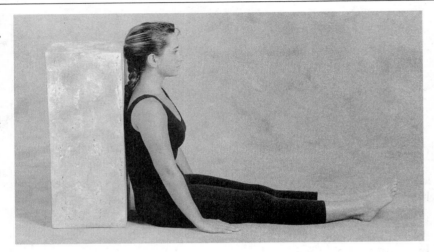

- Place right hand 1 inch above the waist on the muscle to the right side of the spine (muscle will feel firm and ropelike).

  Place left hand behind crease of the right knee.

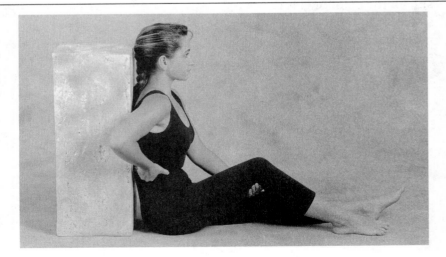

- Right hand stays in the same position.

  Left hand is placed on the center of the back of the right calf. This is just below the fullest part of the calf.

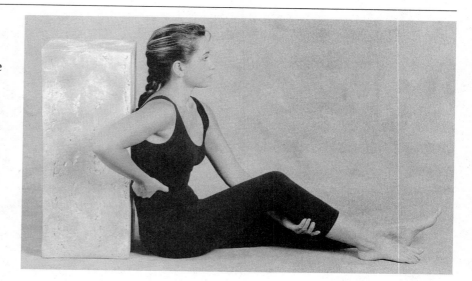

- Right hand remains 1 inch above the waist on the muscle to the side of the spine.

  Left hand is placed just below the ankle bone on the outside of the right heel.

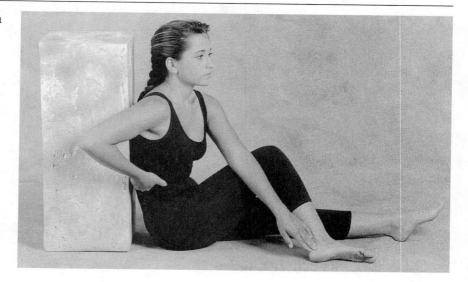

- Right hand remains 1 inch above the waist on the muscle to the side of the spine.

- Left hand holds the front and back of the right little toe at the nail.

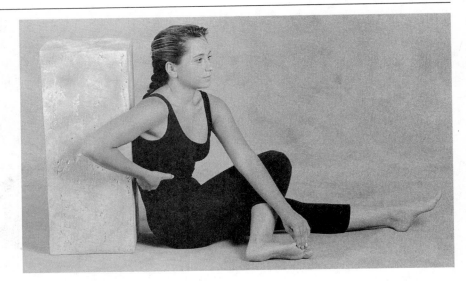

Suggested Reading for Acupressure

The Academy of Traditional Chinese Medicine. *An Outline of Chinese Acupuncture.* New York: Pergamon Press, 1975.

Bauer, C. *Acupressure for Women.* Freedom, CA: The Crossing Press, 1987.

Chang, S. T. *The Complete Book of Acupuncture.* Berkeley, CA: Celestial Arts, 1976.

Gach, M. R., and C. Marco. *Acu-Yoga.* Tokyo: Japan Publications, 1981

Houston, F. M. *The Healing Benefits of Acupressure.* New Canaan, CT: Keats Publishing, 1974.

Kenyon, J. *Acupressure Techniques.* Rochester, VT: Healing Arts Press, 1980.

Nickel, D. J. *Acupressure for Athletes.* New York: Henry Holt, 1984.

Pendleton, B., and B. Mehling. *Relax With Self-Therap/Ease.* Englewood Cliffs, NJ: Prentice-Hall, 1984.

Teeguarden, I. *Acupressure Way of Health: Jin Shin Do.* Tokyo: Japan Publications, 1978.

12

Treating Menstrual Cramps with Drugs

Women use many different types of medications to treat menstrual cramps. Some of these products can be bought over the counter, while other, stronger drugs need a doctor's prescription. Some medications—such as narcotics, diuretics, and muscle relaxants—have been around for a long time and have been the traditional treatments for cramps. Others, specifically the antiprostaglandins, have been widely available for use in treating menstrual cramps only for the past 15 years; these have provided women with a major source of symptom relief.

Over-the-Counter Medications

Many medications for menstrual cramp relief are available over the counter. They tend to be more effective for mild symptoms. My patients have reported to me over the years that these products usually don't provide sufficient relief of the more severe symptoms. One of the oldest cramp relief medications is simply aspirin. Interestingly enough, aspirin is a mild prostaglandin inhibitor, although it's only one-thirtieth as strong as the new antiprostaglandin drugs. Always take aspirin with food to avoid stomach discomfort, and use it with great caution if you have a preexisting peptic ulcer or a tendency toward heartburn, because it can worsen or reactivate symptoms.

Another, more recently available prostaglandin inhibitor is ibuprofen. This drug is sold over the counter as Advil or Nuprin. These products are allowed to be sold without prescription in 200 milligram tablets. The dose commonly used for menstrual cramps is two tablets, or 400 milligrams, taken every six hours. Like aspirin, ibuprofen should be taken with food as it can worsen or cause gastrointestinal upset.

Another group of over-the-counter remedies for menstrual pain contains several drugs used in combination. Products such as Midol, Pamprin, and a number of others on the market contain aspirin, an antispasmodic to relieve muscle tension, caffeine (which causes widening in the diameter of peripheral blood vessels), and sometimes a diuretic for relief of congestive symptoms. Be careful to follow the dosage instructions on the bottle; if used in excess, many of these drugs can cause undesired side effects. As mentioned earlier, aspirin can cause gastric distress. Caffeine can make people nervous and jittery and may also upset the stomach by increasing gastric acid secretion. Diuretics can promote loss of minerals. Another commonly used ingredient in these products is pyrilamine, an antihistamine. Antihistamines are normally used to relieve symptoms of allergy such as nasal congestion. They also have as a side effect the tendency to cause drowsiness or sedation and are used in menstrual remedies for these sedative effects. Although the doses used are small, some women who are unusually sensitive may encounter side effects.

Prescription Medications

Prostaglandin Inhibitors. These drugs, which are also called nonsteroidal anti-inflammatory agents, are a relatively new class of drugs being used for the treatment of menstrual cramps. They tend to be very effective in relieving the symptoms of primary spasmodic dysmenorrhea and, for many women, can make the difference between being able to function during the menstrual period or being incapacitated by pain and spending one to two days in bed. Antiprostaglandins are also used effectively to treat the pain symptoms in women with endometriosis, a common cause of secondary dysmenorrhea. These medications are particularly useful since they have both anti-inflammatory and painkilling activity. Originally developed for the treatment of arthritis, they primarily available by prescription. They include Motrin, Naprosyn, Anaprox, and Ponstel. Ibuprofen (Advil, Nuprin) is available in higher dosage levels as Motrin. These drugs must be used carefully, however, since they can cause gastrointestinal bleeding and peptic ulcer disease, or even reactivate a preexisting ulcer. Approximately 10 percent of women who use these medications report digestive symptoms. Symptoms including heartburn, nausea, vomiting, diarrhea, constipation, and poor digestion can occur as the result of using these medications. To lessen the likelihood of these side effects, only take these medications with food and report any significant digestive symptoms to your physician. Some women report other unpleasant symptoms when using prostaglandin inhibitors, such as drowsiness, headaches, vertigo, dizziness, rashes, blurred vision, anemia, edema, and heart palpitations. Avoid using these drugs with aspirin, since both can cause gastrointestinal bleeding and irritation.

Narcotics. Narcotics such as codeine are very effective painkillers and can certainly numb the discomfort of menstrual cramps or endometriosis. They do, however, have significant side effects and don't reverse the underlying cause of the menstrual cramps or halt the spread of endometrial implants. These side effects commonly include constipation, nausea, and drowsiness. Be sure to avoid driving your car when using a significant painkiller because you may fall asleep at the wheel. Other painkillers like Darvon or relaxants like Valium are also prescribed. Although Valium is an effective relaxant, it can also cause drowsiness and sedation. All of these drugs can cause addiction. Women often find that higher doses and more frequent usage is needed to create a beneficial therapeutic effect if these drugs are used on a habitual basis.

I generally recommend that these drugs be used only on a very infrequent basis and only if symptoms are particularly severe.

Diuretics.   Drugs such as HydroDiuril or Hygroton are strong medications usually prescribed to treat the fluid retention symptoms of primary congestive dysmenorrhea. Though diuretics help to relieve bloating and fluid weight gain by increasing fluid loss through the urinary tract, they also increase the loss of important minerals such as potassium and calcium from the body. Over time, potassium depletion can become a significant problem with frequent diuretic use. Side effects of potassium loss include weakness, fatigue, poor physical stamina, and muscle twitching and immobility. I used to see this problem much more commonly in the 1970s than now, since diuretic use has decreased with the advent of the new antiprostaglandin drugs. If you use any diuretic, be sure to increase your intake of fresh fruits, vegetables, and raw seeds and nuts, which are excellent sources of essential minerals. Eating a banana or two a day is particularly advised. It is easy to digest and contains a lot of potassium.

Birth Control Pills.   These drugs prevent ovulation and thereby decrease the progesterone and prostaglandin accumulation during the second half of the menstrual cycle. This buildup of these two hormones has been associated with menstrual cramps. I recommend the birth control pills most strongly for women who wish to use this method as their primary form of contraception. Otherwise, a woman is using hormonal therapy all month to treat one or two days per month of menstrual cramp symptoms. With endometriosis, however, the use of hormonal therapy has been an important treatment. Continuous hormonal therapy helps to relieve menstrual pain, however, it does not reverse the buildup of endometrial implants. There are women, however, who should avoid using birth control pills because of possible adverse side effects. These include women with a history of liver or gall bladder disease, migraine headaches, high blood pressure, and blood clots in the legs or pelvis. If you are interested in using the birth control pill, check with your physician to see if you are a good candidate.

Other Hormonal Therapies. Other hormonal therapies have also been used effectively to suppress estrogen and therefore menstruation. Two types of drugs are currently in use: synthetic steroids or hormones such as Danazol, and synthetic derivatives of the gonadotropin-releasing hormone (GnRH) such as Lupron. Danazol is a derivative of testosterone, the male hormone. It acts on the pituitary, the master endocrine gland, to inhibit hormonal output and suppress ovulation. Danazol is very effective in dissolving small endometrial implants and helps relieve symptoms in 85 percent of women who use it.

There are, however, significant drawbacks to its use. Twenty percent of women who take Danazol experience the recurrence of endometriosis symptoms within a year after stopping the drug. This percentage tends to increase with time. Danazol also causes masculinizing side effects such as acne, decrease in breast size, weight gain, oiliness of the skin and hair, deepening of the voice, and enlargement of the clitoris. Other side effects may be the same as those experienced in menopause due to the low levels of estrogen caused by the drug's therapeutic effects. These include hot flashes, increased sweating, and vaginal dryness. Obviously Danazol is a powerful drug that should be taken only after careful discussion between you and your physician.

Lupron, a commonly used gonadotropin releasing factor, is also an effective drug therapy for endometriosis. As many as 70 percent of women using Lupron or other drugs of this type note rapid symptom relief. Lupron is also used to shrink fibroid tumors. Unlike Danazol, Lupron does not cause masculinizing side effects, but does cause a marked pseudomenopause because of significantly lowered estrogen levels. Like Danazol, Lupron can cause women to experience hot flashes, vaginal dryness, and a decrease in sex drive. Other side effects have included anemia, bone pain, nausea, vomiting, edema, low blood pressure, and sleep disorders. As with using Danazol, endometriosis symptoms may reoccur once the Lupron is stopped, just as they can reoccur after discontinuing Danazol. A woman can be back where she started before instituting the hormonal therapy.

If your secondary dysmenorrhea has another cause, such as pelvic inflammatory disease (PID), this situation must be treated in order to prevent recurrent pelvic pain. In this case, your physician should prescribe the appropriate antibiotic to destroy the infective agent. If drug therapy is unable to halt the severity of painful symptoms due to the structural damage and scarring that PID causes, a woman may need to undergo a complete hysterectomy to finally gain adequate pain relief.

Medications for Cramps

Over-the-Counter Medications
Aspirin
Ibuprofen (Advil, Nuprin)
Midol
Pamprin

Prescription Drugs

Antiprostaglandin Inhibitors
Motrin
Anaprox
Ponstel
Naprosyn

Narcotics
Codeine
Darvon

Relaxants
Valium

Diuretics
HydroDiuril
Hygroton

Hormonal Therapies
Birth control pills
Danazol
Lupron

13

How to Put Your Program Together

Menstrual Cramps—A Self Help Program has given you a complete self help program to help prevent and relieve your symptoms. The Complete Treatment Chart on page 62 summarizes the many treatment options presented in this book. This chart should be very helpful to refer to as you put your own program together. Try the treatment options that feel most comfortable to you. You may find, for example, in trying the exercises or stress reduction techniques, that certain routines feel better to you than others. If that is the case, practice the ones that bring you the greatest sense of relief for your particular symptoms.

Don't get bogged down in details. Always keep in mind that your ultimate goal is relief of your menstrual cramps and a general improvement in your overall health and well-being. I generally recommend beginning any self help program slowly so that you can get used to the lifestyle changes in a comfortable manner. People differ in their abilities to adjust to major lifestyle changes. Though some of my patients like to eliminate their old, unhealthy habits as quickly as possible, many other women find such rapid changes in their long-term habits to be too stressful. Find the pace that works for you.

Enjoy the program. I always tell my patients to regard their self help program as an enjoyable adventure. The exercise and stress-reduction programs should give you a sense of energy and well-being. The menus and food selections I've recommended in this book provide you with an opportunity to try delicious and healthful new foods.

As you do the program, don't set up unrealistic or too strict expectations for yourself. You don't have to be perfect to get great results. Just follow the guidelines of the program as best you can and as your schedule permits.

It is not a disaster if you forget to take your vitamins occasionally or don't have time to exercise on any particular day. Don't be discouraged if you can't follow the dietary recommendations on vacations, holidays, and birthdays. Periodically, review the guidelines outlined in this book and continue to adapt your lifestyle to the healthful suggestions that I've shared with you from my years of medical practice. Over time you will notice many beneficial changes.

Be your own feedback system. Your own body will tell you if you are on the right track and if what you are doing is making you feel better. It will also tell you if your current diet and emotional stresses are worsening your symptoms. Remember that even moderate changes in your habits can make significant differences.

The Menstrual Cramps Workbook

Fill out the workbook section of this book. The workbook questionnaires will help you to evaluate which areas in your life have contributed the most to your symptoms and which areas need the most work. Use the workbook every month or two as you follow the self-help program. The workbook will help you to see the areas in which you are making the most progress, both with symptom relief and the initiation of healthier lifestyle habits. The workbook can help give you feedback in an organized and easy-to-use manner.

Diet and Nutritional Supplements

I recommend that you make all nutritional changes gradually. Many women find breakfast the easiest meal to change because it is simple and often eaten at home. To change your other meals and snacks, I recommend that you periodically review the list of foods to eliminate and foods to emphasize provided in this book. Each month pick a few foods that you are willing to eliminate from your diet. Try replacing them with the foods that help to prevent and relieve menstrual cramps, low back pain, and congestive symptoms. The recipes and menus that I've included in this book should be very helpful. The menus can provide you with helpful guidelines as you restructure your own needs.

Vitamins, minerals, and herbal supplements can help to complete your nutritional needs and speed up the healing process. For most women, they are a very important part of their program.

Stress-Reduction and Breathing Exercises

The stress-reduction and breathing exercises play an important role in facilitating the physical healing process. I find that all my patients heal more rapidly from almost any problem when they are calm, happy, and relaxed. Some of the exercises also provide a number of important visualizations that actually help you set a blueprint in your mind for optimal health. This allows the body and mind to work together in harmony.

Begin the program by putting 15 minutes to a half-hour aside each day, depending on the flexibility of your schedule. Try all the stress-reduction and breathing exercises listed in this book. Choose the combination that works best for you. Practice stress management on a regular basis and be aware of your habitual breathing patterns. Both of these techniques will help retrain your uterine, pelvic, and back muscles so that you can go through your period in a comfortable manner.

You do not need to spend enormous amounts of time on these exercises. Many women are too busy to spend an hour a day meditating. Even ten minutes out of your daily schedule can be helpful. You may find that the quietest times for you are early in the morning before you get out of bed and late at night before going to sleep. Other women simply choose to take a break during the day. You can close the door to your office or go into your bedroom at home for ten minutes to relax. Use the time to breathe deeply, do the visualizations, or meditate. You will be much calmer and more relaxed afterward.

Exercise

Moderate exercise should be done on a regular basis, at least three times a week. Aerobic exercise can help to improve both circulation and oxygenation to tight, constricted muscles, thereby helping you to relax. It is important, however, to do your exercise routine in a slow, comfortable manner. Frenetic exercise that is too fast-paced can push your muscles to the point of exhaustion and actually tense them further. It is important that women with menstrual cramps and low back pain keep their muscles and joints flexible and supple. Try the fitness and flexibility exercises in this book.

To do the stretches and acupressure exercises described in this book, I recommend that you set aside a half-hour each day for the first week or two of starting your self help program. Try all the exercises. After an initial period of exploration, choose the ones that you enjoy the most and that seem to give you the most relief. Practice them on a regular basis so that they can help to prevent and reduce your symptoms.

Conclusion

I wish to reaffirm that each of us can do a tremendous amount for ourselves to assure optimal health and well-being. By having access to information, education, and health resources, every woman can play a major role in creating her own state of good health. Practice the beneficial self help techniques that I've outlined in this book. Follow good nutritional habits, exercise, and practice regular stress reduction techniques.

By combining good principles of self-care along with your regular medical care, you can enjoy the same wonderful results that my patients and I have had for a life of good health and well-being.

Index

Abdominal muscles
    acupressure, 183
    breathing, 145
    physical, 164–65
    stress, 131
    yoga, 172, 174, 175
Acorn squash, 100
ACTH, 14
Acupressure, 62, 183–98, 208
Acupuncture meridians, 157
Advil, 200
Aerobic exercises, 154, 208
Affirmations, 137–38
Alcohol, 73–74
    substitution for, 80
Alkaline bath 140
Almond milk, 89
Amino acid, 112
Angelica sinensis, 113
Ankles, joint motion and flex-
        ibility, 157
Anti-inflammatory agents, 200–01
Anti-inflammatory herbs, 113–14
Antihistamine, 200
Antiprostaglandins, 201, 202
Anxiety, relief of, 194–95
Apple with almond butter, 105

Applesauce, spread, 93
Asparagus, 99
Aspirin, 113, 114, 199–200
Autonomic nervous system, 147

Back muscle exercise, 161–62
Back pain
    relief of, 132, 133, 148, 161, 166,
        169, 170, 172, 174, 175,
        176, 180, 185, 196–98
Back twist, 167–68
Banana, 85, 105
Bath
    alkaline, 140
    hydrogen peroxide, 140–41
Bean, 86, 94
Beet salad, 97
Biofeedback therapy, 141–42
Birth control pill, 109, 202–03
Black cohosh, 113
Black currant oil, 116
Black haw, 113
Bloating, 189–92
Blood-circulation enhancers,
        114–15
Borage oil, 116
Bran, 65

Bread, whole grain, 66
Breakfast
    menus, 85
    recipes, 88–93
Breathing exercise, 62
    color with golden light, 152
    color with red and blue,
        151–52
    deep abdominal, 146
    emotional cleansing, 150
    grounding, 148–49
    muscle tension release, 149–50
    peaceful slow, 147–48
Broccoli, 99
Brown rice, 85, 86, 92, 98
Butter
    almond, 105
    sesame, 105
    substitute flax oil for, 77–78

Caffeine, 75, 78, 200
Cake, rice
    with nut butter and jam, 104
    with tuna fish, 105
Calcium salad, 96
Calcium, 64
    food sources of, 124
    nutrition of, 110
Carob, 78, 81
Carrot soup, 95
Carrot, steamed, 100
Cauliflower, 99
Cereal
    brown rice, 92
    instant flax, 90
    millet, 64–65, 91
    tofu, 90
    whole grain, 65
Chamomile, 112, 113
Cheese, substitution of, 76–77
Chi, 183

Chocolate, 78–79, 81
Codeine, 201
Coffee, 78, 81
Cole slaw, 98
Color breathing
    with golden light, 152
    with red and blue, 151–52
Concentrated sweeteners, 79
Congestive dysmenorrhea, 14–15
Corn muffins, 93
Corpus luteum, 11
Crackers, 66

Dairy products
    avoidance of, 71–72
    substitution for, 76–77
Danazol, 203, 204
Darvon, 201, 204
Decaffeinated, 78
Deep abdominal breathing, 146
Depression, 176
    relief of, 194
Diet supplements, 207
Dietary principles, 63–80
Dinner
    menus, 86–87
    recipes, 94–105
Diuretic herbs, 114
Diuretics, 199, 200
Dizziness, 108, 111
Dong Quai, 113
Dysmenorrhea. See Menstrual
        cramps.

Eating habits, 46–49
Electromagnetic energy, 183
Emotional state, 55–56, 150. See
        also Stress.
Endometriosis, 17, 201, 202, 203, 204
Endometrium, 10, 17
Essential fatty acids, 115–17

Estrogen, 11, 13, 16, 203
Evening primrose oil, 116
Exercises, 50
    acupressure, 183–98
    breathing, 145–52, 207
    self help program for, 207
    for stress reduction, 131–43,
        207–8
    yoga, 169–81

Faintness, 108, 111
Fallopian tube, 11
Fatigue, 108, 109, 111, 113, 169, 176
    relief of, 194–95
Fats, 72
Fatty acids, 13–14
    food sources of, 123
Fertilization, 11
Fiber, 65
Fibroid tumors, 16
Fish oil, 117
Fish, 69–70
    food sources of, 121–25
Fitness
    exercises, 156–68
    general, 155
    performance of, 155–56
Flax cereal, 90
Flax shake, 89
Flax oil, 116, 117
    with popcorn, 105
    substitution for butter, 77–78
    with vegetables, 99, 100
Flax seed, 116
Flax spread, 93
Flexibility, 156–60
Flour, 80
Fluid retention, 189–92
Focusing exercise, 133
Follicle-stimulating hormones
        (FSH), 10–11

Food allergies, 14–15
Food sources
    of essential fatty acids, 123
    of minerals, 121, 124–25
    of vitamins, 120, 122–23
Food, 63–64
    avoidance of, 70–75
    eating habits for, 46–49
    healthy substitution for, 64–70
Fruit, 67–68
    food sources of, 121, 125
    substitution for sugar, 79

Gamma linolenic acid, 115–16
Ginger, 114
Ginkgo biloba, 115
Gluten, 64–65
Gonadotropin, 203
Grain, 64–67, 80
    food sources of, 120–25
    starches, 98–99
Green beans and almonds, 100

Herbs, 62, 73, 78, 88
    and acupressure, 183
    for menstrual cramps, 112–15
    of teas, 88, 114
Hops, 112, 113
Hips, joint motion and flexibility,
    159–60
Hormonal therapy, 203–4
Hummus, 101
HydroDiuril, 202, 204
Hydrogen peroxide bath, 140–41
Hydrotherapy, 140–41
Hygroton, 202, 204

Ibuprofen, 200, 204
Iron
    food sources of, 121
    nutrition of, 111

Joint motion, 156–60

Kale, steamed, 100
Kasha, 98
Knees, joint motion and flex-
    ibility, 158

Leg muscle tension, 161–62
Legumes
    dietary principles for, 66–67
    food sources of, 120–21
Life energy, 183–84
Linoleic, 115–17
Linolenic, 115–17
Low back release, 166
Low back twist, 167
Lower back arch, 163
Lower back, 61–62
    focusing of, 133
    relief of, 161, 166, 167, 171,
        173–78, 180, 185–88,
        193, 196–97
    stretching of, 163, 166, 167,
        173–78
    treatment chart for, 62
Lunch
    menus, 86–87
    recipes, 94–105
Lupron, 203–4
Luteinizing hormones (LH), 11

Magnesium salad, 96
Magnesium, 64
    food sources of, 125
    nutrition of, 111
Main dishes, 101–4
Meal plans, 85–87
Meat, 69–70
    food sources of, 120–25
Medications
    over-the-counter, 199–200, 204

prescription, 200–204
Meditation
    healing, 135–36
    peaceful, 136–37
Menstrual cramps, 9–10
    acupressure for, 183–98
    breathing exercises for, 145–52
    dietary principles for, 63–81
    evaluating symptoms of, 21–45
    medications for, 199–204
    menus, meal plans, and
        recipes for, 83–105
    physical exercises for, 153–68
    risk factors for, 18, 46–57
    stress reduction for, 51–56,
        131–43
    treatment chart for, 62
    types of, 12–18
    vitamins, minerals, and herbs
        for, 107–25
    workbook for, 21–56
    yoga for, 169–81
Menstrual cycle, 10–11
Menus, 85–87
Meridians, 183–84
Midol, 200
Milk breakfast shake, 88
Milk, replacement in, 76–77
Millet cereal, 64, 65, 91
Minerals, 110–11
    food sources for, 121, 124, 125
    supplements for, 119, 207
Muffins, corn, 93
Muscle relaxing, 50, 134–35
    herbs, 113
Muscle tension, 133–35, 141–42,
    149–50, 161
Music, 141

Narcotics, 201–2
Nausea, relief of, 193

Niacin, 108–9
Nonalcoholic, 74, 80
Nondairy milk, 88
Normal menstrual cycle, 10–11
Nuprin, 200
Nutrition
    dietary principles for, 63–81
    guidelines, 46–56
    risk factors for, 46–49
    supplements for, 117–25, 207
    treatment chart for, 62
Nuts and seeds, 68–69
    food sources of, 121–23, 125

Oatmeal and rice pancakes, 92
Oats, 64, 65
Oils, 70
    food sources of, 123
Oriental herbs, 113–14, 183
Ovaries, 11
Ovulation, 11

Pain, low back, 132, 133, 148–49,
        169, 173
Pamprin, 200
Pancakes, 66, 92
Parasympathic system, 147
Passionflower, 112
Pasta, 66, 102
Pea soup, 96
Pelvic inflammatory disease,
        16–17, 204
Pelvic, 148, 161–62
    arch, 172
    congestion of, 169, 174
    exercise of, 167–68
Peony root, 113
Pesto, 102
Physical exercise, 62, 153–68
PID, 16–17
Pituitary, 11

Popcorn, 105
Potassium, 64, 79
    depletion of, 202
Potato
    baked, 199
    milk, 77
    salad, 97
    soup, 96
Poultry, 69–70
    food sources of, 120–25
Prescriptions, 200–204
Primary congestive dysmenorrhea,
        14–15, 18
Primary spasmodic dysmenorrhea,
        12–14, 18
Progesterone, 11, 12, 13
Prostaglandin inhibitors
    over-the-counter, 199–200
    prescription, 200–201
Prostaglandins, 13–14, 109, 115, 116
Pumpkin seed oil, 116, 117
Pyrilamine, 200
Pyridoxine, 109

Recipes, 83–84, 88–105
    healthy ingredients for, 75–81
Relaxant herb, 113
Relaxation
    abdominal, 164–65
    biofeedback, 141–42
    exercises, 132, 133–38
    hydrotherapy, 140–41
    low back, 166
    music, 141
    tension, 161–62
Reproductive system, exercise
    balance of, 185–88
Rice, 64, 65, 66
    brown, 98
    cake, 104
    cereal, 92

pancakes, 92
pesto, 102
tofu, 101, 102
Risk factors, 15, 18–19, 46–56
Rye, 64, 65, 66

Salad
    beet, 97
    cole slaw, 98
    potato, 97
    spinach, 97
    vegetable, 96
Salicin, 113
Salmon, poached, 103
Salt, 73
    substitution of, 79–80
Seafood, 69–70
Seaweed, 79
Secondary dysmenorrhea, 16, 18
Sedative herbs, 112–13
Seeds and nuts, 68–69
Self help guideline, 46–56
Self-program, 61–62, 63, 204–9
Serotonin, 112
Sesame milk, 89
Simonton, Carl, 138
Snacks and spreads, 93, 104–5
Sound therapy, 141
Soups
    black bean, 94
    carrot, 95
    split pea and potato, 96
    tomato-lentil, 96
    vegetable, 95
Soy, substitution
    for cheese, 77
    for salt, 79
Spasmodic dysmenorrhea, 12–14
Spine
    joint motion and flexibility,
        156–60

lumbar, 167–68
    stretches, 176–77
Split pea soup, 96
Spouse, 54–55
Spreads, 93, 104–5
Squash, 100
Starches, 98–99
Stir-fry, 103
Stress, 110
    emotional, 131, 132
    evaluation of, 51–56
    exercises, 167–68
    guidelines, 46–56
    reduction, 46, 50, 62, 131–43,
        207–8
Stretches
    lower back, 163, 167–68
    yoga, 169–79
Sugar, 74–75
    substitution of, 79
Sweeteners, 79
Sympathic system, 147

Tabouli, 101
Tacos, vegetable, 103
Tea, herbal, 78, 88, 114
Tension
    abdominal, 164–65, 170
    muscle 133–35, 141–42, 149–50,
        161–62
    release, 149–50

Toes, flexibility and joint motion
    for, 157
Tofu, 66
    almond stir-fry and, 103
    cereal, 90
    dairy substitution for,
        76–77
    pesto and, 102
    rice and, 101, 102
Tomato sauce, 102
Tomato-lentil soup, 96
Trail mix, 104
Treatment chart, 22–45, 62, 205–9
Tryptophan, 112
Tumors, fibroid, 16
Tuna, broiled, 104

Unicorn root, 113
Uterus, 10
    cramping, 156
    fibroid tumor of, 16
    lining of, 10, 11

Valerian root, 112–13
Valium, 201
Vegetables, 67
    food sources, 121–25
    main dishes, 99–100
    for menstrual cramps, 67
    salad, 96
    soup, 95

Visualizations, 138–40
Vitamin B complex
    food sources of, 120
    nutrition of, 66, 108
Vitamin B_3
    nutrition of, 108–9
Vitamin B_6
    food sources of, 122
    nutrition of, 66, 108–9
Vitamin C, 113
    food sources of, 122
    nutrition of, 67–68, 109–10
Vitamin E, 117
    food sources of, 123
    nutrition of, 110
Vitamin, 62, 65
    nutrition of, 108–10
    treatment and prevention of,
        107–10

Weight gain, 189–92
Wheat, avoidance of, 64–65, 80
White willow bark, 113–14
Whole grains, 64–67, 80
Workbook, 22–47, 206

Yin and yang, 112
Yoga, 62, 169–80

Zucchini and eggplant, 100

About Susan M. Lark, M.D.

Susan M. Lark, M.D., is a noted authority on women's health care and preventative medicine. Dr. Lark has been on the clinical faculty of Stanford University Medical School, Division of Family and Community Medicine, where she continues to teach. She has been the director of a number of clinical programs for women and worked with thousands of patients in her twenty years of private practice. Dr. Lark lectures widely on women's health issues and is the author of a series of books published by Celestial Arts including: *PMS Self Help Book, The Menopause Self Help Book, Menstrual Cramps Self Help Book, Fibroid Tumors & Endometriosis Self Help Book, Heavy Menstrual Flow & Anemia Self Help Book, Anxiety & Stress Self Help Book, Chronic Fatigue Self Help Book, The Estrogen Decision Self Help Book,* and *The Women's Health Companion.* She also presents workshops and seminars on women's health issues. If you would like to contact her for more personalized guidance, Dr. Lark is available for phone consultation at (415) 964-7268. She also presents workshops and seminars on women's health issues.

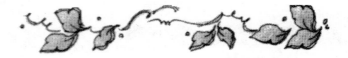

Acknowledgment

The author and publisher wish to extend a special acknowledgment to Shelly Reeves-Smith and Cracom Corporation for permission to reproduce the creative line drawings found in the food section of this book. These and additional drawings, together with a collection of wonderful recipes, may be found in the cookbook *Just a Matter of Thyme* available in your local gift or book store. Inquires may be addressed to Among Friends, P.O. Box 1476, Camdenton, MO 65020 or call toll free (800) 377-3566.

Dr. Susan Lark's
Complete Self Help Library on Women's Health

❦ Heavy Menstrual Flow & Anemia

One in five American women suffers from anemia due to iron or folic acid deficiency. Dr. Lark helps you understand and identify the causes, symptoms, and diagnosis of anemia, as well as heavy and irregular menstrual bleeding. Assess your symptoms and begin your own natural self help treatment. —*164 pages*

❦ Anxiety & Stress

Millions of women suffer from emotional distress, nervous tension, panic, and anxiety...often on a daily basis. Dr. Lark discusses the causes, symptoms, and diagnosis of anxiety and other emotional conditions, and guides you through an effective self help treatment program. —*284 pages*

❦ Chronic Fatigue

Chronic fatigue is one of the most common—and most commonly misunderstood—medical complaints for which women seek their doctors' advice. Dr. Lark has designed programs to help you relieve chronic fatigue syndrome, as well as underlying conditions, including candida, infections, depression, allergies, and fatigue due to PMS, menopause, and thyroid conditions. —*234 pages*

❦ Fibroid Tumors & Endometriosis

Over 40% of American women develop fibroid tumors of the uterus. Endometriosis is common to menstruating women from ages 20 to 45. Both conditions cause a variety of distressing symptoms. Identify the signs, symptoms, and risk factors, and then formulate your own treatment program with Dr. Lark's help. —*264 pages*

❦ Menstrual Cramps

Fifty percent of all women suffer from painful menstrual periods. Some have symptoms so severe that they are unable to cope with their normal daily activities. This valuable book describes types and causes of menstrual pain, helps women evaluate their own symptoms, and presents a comprehensive self help program. —*224 pages*

❦ The Estrogen Decision

Should you use estrogen during and after menopause? Get the facts on the benefits, side effects, and risks of estrogen, progesterone, and hormone replacement therapy (HRT). Dr. Lark discusses the latest information on the issues surrounding menopause, and offers alternative treatments for specific menopausal symptoms. —*316 pages*

❦ Menopause

You don't have to dread menopause. Dr. Lark offers the first completely safe, practical, all-natural master plan for relieving and preventing menopause symptoms including irritability and hot flashes...as well as a plan to help eliminate the long-term risk of osteoporosis and breast and uterine cancer. —*240 pages*

❦ Premenstrual Syndrome

Dr. Lark's plan helps you eliminate the causes of PMS symptoms, including anxiety, pain, weight gain, chocolate cravings, mood swings, depression, bloating, and breast tenderness. Learn how to deal with sugar cravings and caffeine addiction, prevent depression and mood swings, and alleviate pain. —*240 pages*

❦ The Women's Health Companion: Self Help Nutrition Guide and Cookbook

The only cookbook that answers women's special nutritional needs, including recipes to prevent and treat PMS, osteoporosis, breast cancer, heart disease, menopause, fibrocystic breast disease, and endometriosis. Also includes menus and a discussion of how to make an easy transition to your healthy new diet. —*370 pages*